The New Diabetic Diet Cookbook for Seniors Over 60

Lots of Easy, Quick, and Tasty Recipes to Lower Blood Sugar, Increase Energy, and Improve Your Health Without Feeling Like You're on a Diet

Filipo Gaona

© Copyright 2025 by Filipo Gaona - All rights reserved.

The purpose of this text is to present accurate and trustworthy information on the facts and topic covered. from a policy statement that was equally accepted and authorized by an American Bar Association committee and a committee of associations and publishers.

This text may not be reproduced, duplicated, or distributed in any way, whether in print or electronic format. All rights protected.

Since all of the material presented here is accurate and consistent, the recipient and reader bear full responsibility for any liability resulting from the use or abuse of any procedures, guidelines, or directions in this document, whether due to negligence or other causes. In no event will the publication be held accountable for any recovery, damages, or monetary loss that can be directly or indirectly linked to the material presented here.

Each author is the owner of any copyrights not owned by the publisher.

Since the material presented here is intended solely for informative purposes, it can be applied broadly. The information is provided without any type of contract or guarantee.

Unauthorized use of trademarks occurs, when trademarks are published without the owner's consent or approval. The brands and trademarks in this book are all owned by their respective owners and are solely used for illustration purposes; they are not associated with this book.

Table of Content

INTRODUCTION 7

INTRODUCTION 7

    UNDERSTANDING DIABETES AND ITS IMPACT ON YOUR HEALTH 7

    UNDERSTANDING DIABETES AND ITS IMPACT ON YOUR HEALTH 7

    THE IMPORTANCE OF NUTRITION FOR SENIORS LIVING WITH DIABETES 9

    THE IMPORTANCE OF NUTRITION FOR SENIORS LIVING WITH DIABETES 9

    KEY TERMS AND CONCEPTS: GLYCEMIC INDEX, CARB COUNTING, PORTION CONTROL 10

    KEY TERMS AND CONCEPTS: GLYCEMIC INDEX, CARB COUNTING, PORTION CONTROL 10

CHAPTER 1: GETTING STARTED WITH A STRUCTURED EATING PLAN 12

CHAPTER 1: GETTING STARTED WITH A STRUCTURED EATING PLAN 12

    THE 30-DAY MEAL PLAN: HOW IT WORKS 12

    THE 30-DAY MEAL PLAN: HOW IT WORKS 12

    TIPS FOR MEAL PREP AND GROCERY SHOPPING ON A BUDGET 14

    TIPS FOR MEAL PREP AND GROCERY SHOPPING ON A BUDGET 14

    HOW TO CREATE A BALANCED PLATE FOR BLOOD SUGAR CONTROL 15

    HOW TO CREATE A BALANCED PLATE FOR BLOOD SUGAR CONTROL 15

CHAPTER 2: ENERGIZING BREAKFASTS TO START YOUR DAY RIGHT 17

CHAPTER 2: ENERGIZING BREAKFASTS TO START YOUR DAY RIGHT 17

    Cinnamon-Spiced Chia & Flaxseed Pudding 17

    Savory Cottage Cheese & Avocado Toast on Sprouted Grain Bread 18

    Pumpkin Pie Oatmeal with Walnuts & Greek Yogurt 18

    Egg & Spinach Breakfast Muffins 19

    Blueberry Almond Flour Pancakes 19

    Zucchini & Cheddar Omelet Roll-Ups 20

    Chia & Hemp Seed Protein Smoothie 20

    Baked Apple & Oatmeal Cups 21

    Avocado & Smoked Salmon Scramble 21

    Coconut & Pecan Overnight Oats 22

    Cauliflower & Cheese Breakfast Hash 22

    Flaxseed & Almond Butter Breakfast Bars 23

Mushroom & Feta Breakfast Wrap 23

Vanilla Ricotta & Berry Parfait 24

Savory Sweet Potato & Egg Bowl 24

Green Power Breakfast Scramble (Kale, Eggs & Turkey Sausage) 25

Sugar-Free Banana Walnut Muffins 25

Spiced Quinoa Breakfast Bowl with Almonds & Coconut Milk 26

Creamy Peanut Butter & Chia Toast on Whole Grain Rye 26

Golden Turmeric Smoothie with Greek Yogurt & Almond Milk 27

CHAPTER 3: FLAVORFUL LUNCHES FOR BALANCED BLOOD SUGAR 28

CHAPTER 3: FLAVORFUL LUNCHES FOR BALANCED BLOOD SUGAR 28

Grilled Lemon Herb Chicken with Quinoa & Roasted Veggies 28

Spinach & Feta Stuffed Portobello Mushrooms 29

Zesty Black Bean & Avocado Salad with Lime Dressing 29

Cauliflower Rice Stir-Fry with Tofu & Sesame Ginger Sauce 30

Mediterranean Chickpea & Cucumber Wrap with Tahini Sauce 30

Baked Salmon with Garlic Butter & Asparagus 31

Spicy Turkey & Zucchini Meatballs with Tomato Basil Sauce 31

Roasted Sweet Potato & Kale Salad with Walnuts & Feta 32

Tuna & White Bean Salad with Olive Oil & Lemon 32

Hearty Lentil & Spinach Soup with Turmeric 33

Grilled Shrimp & Avocado Salad with Cilantro Dressing 33

Cottage Cheese & Cucumber Lettuce Wraps 34

Balsamic Chicken & Roasted Brussels Sprouts 34

Sautéed Garlic Tofu & Bok Choy over Brown Rice 35

Creamy Avocado & Chicken Salad on Whole Grain Toast 35

Beef & Broccoli Stir-Fry with Tamari Sauce 36

Quinoa & Roasted Red Pepper Stuffed Peppers 36

Spinach & Ricotta Zucchini Roll-Ups 37

Almond-Crusted Tilapia with Steamed Green Beans 37

Greek Yogurt & Dill Egg Salad on Whole Wheat Crackers 38

CHAPTER 4: NOURISHING DINNERS FOR MAXIMUM SATISFACTION 39

CHAPTER 4: NOURISHING DINNERS FOR MAXIMUM SATISFACTION..........39

- Garlic Butter Baked Cod with Roasted Brussels Sprouts..........39
- Lemon Herb Grilled Chicken with Cauliflower Mash..........40
- Spaghetti Squash with Turkey Bolognese..........40
- Balsamic Glazed Salmon with Sautéed Spinach..........41
- Stuffed Bell Peppers with Quinoa & Ground Turkey..........41
- Zucchini Noodles with Pesto & Grilled Shrimp..........42
- Slow Cooker Chicken & Vegetable Stew..........42
- Cauliflower Crust Pizza with Tomato & Mozzarella..........43
- Beef & Mushroom Stir-Fry with Tamari Sauce..........43
- Mediterranean Baked Eggplant with Feta & Olives..........44
- Herb-Roasted Chicken Thighs with Garlic Green Beans..........44
- Lentil & Sweet Potato Curry with Coconut Milk..........44
- Parmesan-Crusted Tilapia with Roasted Broccoli..........45
- Spinach & Ricotta Stuffed Chicken Breast..........46
- Grilled Portobello Mushrooms with Garlic & Parmesan..........46
- Cauliflower Fried Rice with Shrimp & Scrambled Egg..........47
- Turkey & Zucchini Meatloaf with Mashed Cauliflower..........47
- Cabbage Stir-Fry with Ground Turkey & Ginger..........48
- Creamy Avocado & Chicken Zoodle Bowl..........48
- Roasted Butternut Squash & Kale Bowl with Quinoa..........49

CHAPTER 5: DELICIOUS SIDES AND VEGETABLES THAT SUPPORT HEALTHY BLOOD SUGAR..........50

CHAPTER 5: DELICIOUS SIDES AND VEGETABLES THAT SUPPORT HEALTHY BLOOD SUGAR..........50

- Garlic Roasted Brussels Sprouts with Almonds..........50
- Sautéed Zucchini & Mushrooms with Parmesan..........51
- Balsamic Glazed Roasted Carrots & Onions..........51
- Spicy Cauliflower Rice with Cilantro & Lime..........52
- Creamy Avocado & Cucumber Salad with Lemon Dressing..........52
- Roasted Sweet Potato Wedges with Paprika..........53
- Sautéed Kale with Garlic & Olive Oil..........53
- Grilled Asparagus with Lemon & Feta..........54
- Herb-Roasted Butternut Squash with Walnuts..........54
- Steamed Green Beans with Toasted Sesame Seeds..........55

- Mashed Cauliflower with Garlic & Chives..55
- Spaghetti Squash with Basil & Cherry Tomatoes..56
- Crispy Baked Eggplant Slices with Italian Herbs...56
- Broccoli & Cheddar Stuffed Mushrooms..57
- Mediterranean Cucumber & Chickpea Salad...57

CHAPTER 6: GUILT-FREE DESSERTS TO SATISFY YOUR SWEET TOOTH..58

CHAPTER 6: GUILT-FREE DESSERTS TO SATISFY YOUR SWEET TOOTH..58

- Dark Chocolate & Almond Butter Chia Pudding..58
- Baked Cinnamon Apples with Walnuts & Greek Yogurt...59
- Coconut Flour Blueberry Muffins..59
- Sugar-Free Chocolate Avocado Mousse...60
- Almond Flour Peanut Butter Cookies...60
- No-Bake Coconut & Chia Energy Bites...61
- Lemon Ricotta Cheesecake Bars...61
- Raspberry & Dark Chocolate Frozen Yogurt Bark..62
- Vanilla Chia & Flaxseed Pudding with Berries...62
- Spiced Pumpkin & Pecan Mug Cake...63
- Chocolate Zucchini Brownies (Low-Carb)...63
- Sugar-Free Banana & Walnut Ice Cream..64
- Toasted Almond & Coconut Macaroons...64
- Strawberry & Basil Greek Yogurt Parfait..65
- Low-Carb Cheesecake with Almond Crust..65

CHAPTER 7: SMART SNACKS TO KEEP YOUR ENERGY UP BETWEEN MEALS......................................66

CHAPTER 7: SMART SNACKS TO KEEP YOUR ENERGY UP BETWEEN MEALS......................................66

- Spicy Roasted Chickpeas with Paprika...66
- Greek Yogurt & Cucumber Dip with Whole Grain Crackers..67
- Almond Butter & Celery Sticks with Chia Seeds..67
- Hard-Boiled Eggs with Avocado & Hot Sauce..68
- Sugar-Free Trail Mix with Nuts & Dark Chocolate Bits..68
- Baked Zucchini Chips with Parmesan..69
- Cottage Cheese & Berries with Flaxseeds..69

Cucumber & Turkey Roll-Ups with Mustard 70

Roasted Pumpkin Seeds with Sea Salt & Cinnamon 70

Mini Bell Peppers Stuffed with Hummus 71

Almond Flour Cheddar Crackers 71

Chia & Coconut Protein Bites 72

Smoked Salmon & Cream Cheese Cucumber Bites 72

Sugar-Free Peanut Butter Protein Bars 73

Sautéed Mushrooms & Spinach on Whole Grain Toast 73

CONCLUSION **74**

CONCLUSION **74**

How to Maintain Long-Term Success with Your Diabetic-Friendly Diet 74

How to Maintain Long-Term Success with Your Diabetic-Friendly Diet 74

The Benefits of Consistency and Planning for Your Health 75

The Benefits of Consistency and Planning for Your Health 75

Encouragement for Your Ongoing Journey to Better Health 76

Encouragement for Your Ongoing Journey to Better Health 76

Introduction

Food shapes health in ways that go far beyond calories and taste. For seniors managing diabetes, every meal is an opportunity to stabilize blood sugar, boost energy, and prevent complications. But eating well isn't just about cutting sugar—it's about understanding how different foods interact with the body, how portion sizes influence glucose levels, and how simple adjustments can make a major difference. Nutrition isn't a set of restrictions; it's a powerful tool for taking control of long-term well-being.

Understanding Diabetes and Its Impact on Your Health

Diabetes isn't just about sugar. It's a condition that reshapes how your body handles energy, affecting everything from your circulation to your brain function. At its core, diabetes is a metabolic disorder where the body either doesn't produce enough insulin or can't use it effectively. Insulin, the hormone responsible for shuttling glucose from the bloodstream into cells for energy, is like a key that unlocks the door to fuel your body. When that system falters, sugar lingers in the blood, leading to a cascade of health issues that can touch nearly every organ.

For seniors over 60, diabetes takes on another layer of complexity. The body's metabolism naturally slows with age, muscle mass declines, and cells become less responsive to insulin—a condition known as insulin resistance. These factors make blood sugar management more delicate, requiring a more intentional approach to diet and lifestyle. Even those who have spent a lifetime without health issues may find themselves dealing with prediabetes or type 2 diabetes as they age, often without obvious symptoms. This silent nature of diabetes is part of what makes it so dangerous. By the time it's diagnosed, high blood sugar may have already begun to damage the nerves, kidneys, and eyes.

The effects aren't always dramatic at first, but they are cumulative. Elevated blood sugar thickens the blood, making it harder for oxygen and nutrients to reach the extremities. Over time, this impairs circulation, increasing the risk of slow-healing wounds, infections, and even amputations in severe cases. The nervous system is also vulnerable—diabetic neuropathy can cause tingling, burning, or numbness in the hands and feet, which can make something as simple as walking a dangerous task.

The cardiovascular system takes a hit as well. Excess glucose in the bloodstream fuels inflammation and contributes to the formation of arterial plaque, increasing the likelihood of high blood pressure, heart disease, and strokes. It's no coincidence that people with diabetes are at significantly higher risk of heart-related complications.

But the effects aren't just physical. Blood sugar fluctuations can influence mood, memory, and cognitive function. Many seniors with diabetes report experiencing mental fog, difficulty concentrating, or unexplained fatigue. There's even mounting evidence linking diabetes to an increased risk of dementia and Alzheimer's, as prolonged exposure to high blood sugar can impair brain health over time.

This doesn't mean diabetes is an unavoidable sentence to declining health. While the condition requires vigilance, it's also one of the most manageable chronic diseases when approached correctly. The right foods, eaten in the right way, can help stabilize blood sugar and prevent complications. Small daily choices —what's on the plate, how much is eaten, and when—can mean the difference between thriving and merely getting by.

Understanding how diabetes affects the body is the first step in reclaiming control. The next step is learning how to fuel the body in a way that supports stable blood sugar, sustained energy, and long-term well-being.

The Importance of Nutrition for Seniors Living with Diabetes

Food is more than fuel—it's information. Every bite you take sends instructions to your body, telling it how to function, how to heal, and how to regulate itself. For seniors managing diabetes, those instructions become even more critical. Unlike younger adults, whose bodies may still compensate for dietary mistakes, aging shifts the metabolism, alters digestion, and makes blood sugar regulation more delicate. The foods that once worked may now trigger erratic glucose levels, leading to fatigue, inflammation, and long-term complications.

The body's ability to handle carbohydrates changes over time. Muscle mass naturally declines with age, and since muscle tissue plays a major role in glucose absorption, this reduction makes it easier for blood sugar to spike after meals. Additionally, insulin sensitivity decreases, meaning the body has to work harder to process the same amount of carbohydrates. What this means in real life is that the sandwich, pasta, or bowl of cereal that may have seemed harmless at 40 or 50 can now send blood sugar soaring at 65 or 70.

Beyond the numbers, nutrition affects how seniors feel on a daily basis. A well-balanced meal provides steady energy, keeps hunger at bay, and prevents the rollercoaster of high and low blood sugar that leads to dizziness, mood swings, and mental fog. Poor food choices, on the other hand, can trigger a cascade of problems—excess sugar fuels inflammation, which contributes to joint pain, worsens circulation, and weakens the immune system. This is why many seniors with diabetes experience slow wound healing, frequent infections, and a higher risk of cardiovascular issues.

The challenge isn't just knowing what to eat, but how to eat in a way that aligns with the body's changing needs. Metabolism slows with age, so portion sizes matter more than ever. Too little food leads to muscle loss and weakness, while too much—even of healthy foods—can cause blood sugar imbalances. Seniors also tend to absorb certain nutrients less efficiently, meaning even a diet that looks good on paper may still leave gaps in vitamins and minerals like B12, magnesium, and vitamin D—nutrients essential for nerve function, bone health, and energy levels.

Hydration plays a major role as well. Aging dulls the body's thirst signals, making dehydration a silent but serious issue. Many seniors don't realize they're not drinking enough until symptoms appear—fatigue, dizziness, headaches, and even confusion. And when dehydration sets in, blood sugar concentrations rise, worsening diabetic symptoms.

What makes diabetes especially tricky is that there's no one-size-fits-all solution. Each person's body responds differently to foods, meaning the key to success isn't just following generic advice but finding what works for the individual. A diet that supports stable blood sugar isn't about restriction—it's about choosing foods that nourish, satisfy, and work with the body rather than against it. Understanding these shifts allows seniors to adapt, making informed choices that lead to better energy, fewer complications, and a better quality of life.

Key Terms and Concepts: Glycemic Index, Carb Counting, Portion Control

Not all foods affect blood sugar the same way. Two meals with the same number of calories can have drastically different impacts on glucose levels, energy, and hunger. This is why understanding key nutritional concepts like the glycemic index, carb counting, and portion control is essential for anyone managing diabetes. These aren't abstract theories; they're practical tools that can help prevent blood sugar spikes, reduce insulin resistance, and make eating feel less like a gamble and more like a strategy.

The **glycemic index (GI)** measures how quickly a carbohydrate-containing food raises blood sugar. The scale ranges from 0 to 100, with pure glucose sitting at the top. Foods with a high GI, like white bread and processed cereals, cause a rapid surge in blood sugar, followed by an equally fast crash. Low-GI foods, such as lentils, non-starchy vegetables, and whole grains, break down more slowly, providing a steady release of energy without overwhelming the body with excess glucose. But the GI doesn't tell the full story. Factors like fiber, fat, and protein can slow digestion, reducing a food's actual impact on blood sugar. For example, a ripe banana has a moderate glycemic index, but pairing it with peanut butter lowers the overall blood sugar response.

While the glycemic index focuses on **how fast** a food affects blood sugar, **carb counting** focuses on **how much** carbohydrate is being consumed. Every gram of carbohydrate eventually turns into glucose, so tracking intake helps regulate blood sugar. But not all carbs are created equal. A slice of whole-grain bread and a can of soda might contain a similar number of carbs, but their impact on the body is vastly different due to fiber, nutrient content, and digestion speed. The goal isn't to eliminate carbohydrates but to choose quality sources in appropriate amounts.

Portion control adds another layer of precision. Even healthy foods can spike blood sugar if eaten in excess. A serving of brown rice is better than white rice, but a heaping plateful can still push glucose levels too high. Over time, portion sizes have expanded dramatically—restaurant meals are often double or triple what the body actually needs, making it easy to consume too many carbs without realizing it. The stomach's ability to register fullness declines with age, meaning seniors may feel just as hungry after overeating as they would with an appropriate portion. Measuring food, using smaller plates, and being mindful of portion sizes can help recalibrate the body's natural hunger cues and prevent unintentional overeating.

Navigating diabetes through nutrition doesn't have to feel overwhelming or restrictive. By understanding how the body processes carbohydrates, recognizing the impact of portion sizes, and choosing foods that support balanced blood sugar, eating becomes a form of self-care rather than a source of stress. Small, consistent changes build the foundation for better energy, fewer complications, and a healthier, more vibrant life.

Chapter 1: Getting Started with a Structured Eating Plan

Managing diabetes isn't about following a rigid diet—it's about creating a structured, sustainable way of eating that works for your body. A clear plan eliminates guesswork, stabilizes blood sugar, and makes meals both enjoyable and nourishing. With the right approach to meal planning, grocery shopping, and portioning, food becomes a tool for better health rather than a source of stress.

The 30-Day Meal Plan: How It Works

Day	Breakfast	Lunch	Dinner	Snack
Day 1	Cinnamon-Spiced Chia & Flaxseed Pudding	Quinoa & Roasted Red Pepper Stuffed Peppers	Lentil & Sweet Potato Curry with Coconut Milk	Smoked Salmon & Cream Cheese Cucumber Bites
Day 2	Zucchini & Cheddar Omelet Roll-Ups	Cottage Cheese & Cucumber Lettuce Wraps	Beef & Mushroom Stir-Fry with Tamari Sauce	Smoked Salmon & Cream Cheese Cucumber Bites
Day 3	Chia & Hemp Seed Protein Smoothie	Sautéed Garlic Tofu & Bok Choy over Brown Rice	Garlic Butter Baked Cod with Roasted Brussels Sprouts	Cucumber & Turkey Roll-Ups with Mustard
Day 4	Creamy Peanut Butter & Chia Toast	Spinach & Ricotta Zucchini Roll-Ups	Cauliflower Crust Pizza with Tomato & Mozzarella	Chia & Coconut Protein Bites
Day 5	Zucchini & Cheddar Omelet Roll-Ups	Balsamic Chicken & Roasted Brussels Sprouts	Zucchini Noodles with Pesto & Grilled Shrimp	Mini Bell Peppers Stuffed with Hummus
Day 6	Cauliflower & Cheese Breakfast Hash	Cottage Cheese & Cucumber Lettuce Wraps	Mediterranean Baked Eggplant with Feta & Olives	Chia & Coconut Protein Bites
Day 7	Avocado & Smoked Salmon Scramble	Grilled Shrimp & Avocado Salad with Cilantro Dressing	Spinach & Ricotta Stuffed Chicken Breast	Hard-Boiled Eggs with Avocado & Hot Sauce
Day 8	Coconut & Pecan Overnight Oats	Cauliflower Rice Stir-Fry with Tofu & Sesame Ginger Sauce	Beef & Mushroom Stir-Fry with Tamari Sauce	Cottage Cheese & Berries with Flaxseeds
Day 9	Green Power Breakfast Scramble	Creamy Avocado & Chicken Salad on Whole Grain Toast	Cauliflower Fried Rice with Shrimp & Scrambled Egg	Sugar-Free Trail Mix with Nuts & Dark Chocolate Bits
Day	Savory Cottage Cheese & Avocado	Grilled Shrimp & Avocado Salad with	Turkey & Zucchini Meatloaf with Mashed	Baked Zucchini Chips with Parmesan

10	Toast	Cilantro Dressing	Cauliflower	
Day 11	Egg & Spinach Breakfast Muffins	Grilled Shrimp & Avocado Salad with Cilantro Dressing	Cauliflower Crust Pizza with Tomato & Mozzarella	Mini Bell Peppers Stuffed with Hummus
Day 12	Chia & Hemp Seed Protein Smoothie	Grilled Lemon Herb Chicken with Quinoa & Roasted Veggies	Cauliflower Crust Pizza with Tomato & Mozzarella	Chia & Coconut Protein Bites
Day 13	Avocado & Smoked Salmon Scramble	Zesty Black Bean & Avocado Salad with Lime Dressing	Herb-Roasted Chicken Thighs with Garlic Green Beans	Mini Bell Peppers Stuffed with Hummus
Day 14	Spiced Quinoa Breakfast Bowl	Sautéed Garlic Tofu & Bok Choy over Brown Rice	Lemon Herb Grilled Chicken with Cauliflower Mash	Chia & Coconut Protein Bites
Day 15	Zucchini & Cheddar Omelet Roll-Ups	Spinach & Ricotta Zucchini Roll-Ups	Herb-Roasted Chicken Thighs with Garlic Green Beans	Sautéed Mushrooms & Spinach on Whole Grain Toast
Day 16	Vanilla Ricotta & Berry Parfait	Beef & Broccoli Stir-Fry with Tamari Sauce	Spinach & Ricotta Stuffed Chicken Breast	Chia & Coconut Protein Bites
Day 17	Chia & Hemp Seed Protein Smoothie	Mediterranean Chickpea & Cucumber Wrap with Tahini Sauce	Spinach & Ricotta Stuffed Chicken Breast	Cucumber & Turkey Roll-Ups with Mustard
Day 18	Pumpkin Pie Oatmeal with Walnuts & Greek Yogurt	Spinach & Feta Stuffed Portobello Mushrooms	Zucchini Noodles with Pesto & Grilled Shrimp	Sugar-Free Trail Mix with Nuts & Dark Chocolate Bits
Day 19	Sugar-Free Banana Walnut Muffins	Roasted Sweet Potato & Kale Salad with Walnuts & Feta	Cauliflower Crust Pizza with Tomato & Mozzarella	Baked Zucchini Chips with Parmesan
Day 20	Chia & Hemp Seed Protein Smoothie	Sautéed Garlic Tofu & Bok Choy over Brown Rice	Spinach & Ricotta Stuffed Chicken Breast	Roasted Pumpkin Seeds with Sea Salt & Cinnamon
Day 21	Pumpkin Pie Oatmeal with Walnuts & Greek Yogurt	Creamy Avocado & Chicken Salad on Whole Grain Toast	Garlic Butter Baked Cod with Roasted Brussels Sprouts	Cucumber & Turkey Roll-Ups with Mustard
Day 22	Flaxseed & Almond Butter Breakfast Bars	Grilled Shrimp & Avocado Salad with Cilantro Dressing	Turkey & Zucchini Meatloaf with Mashed Cauliflower	Hard-Boiled Eggs with Avocado & Hot Sauce
D	Vanilla Ricotta &	Almond-Crusted Tilapia	Lemon Herb Grilled	Almond Flour

Day 23	Berry Parfait	with Steamed Green Beans	Chicken with Cauliflower Mash	Cheddar Crackers
Day 24	Creamy Peanut Butter & Chia Toast	Creamy Avocado & Chicken Salad on Whole Grain Toast	Cauliflower Fried Rice with Shrimp & Scrambled Egg	Baked Zucchini Chips with Parmesan
Day 25	Green Power Breakfast Scramble	Zesty Black Bean & Avocado Salad with Lime Dressing	Cabbage Stir-Fry with Ground Turkey & Ginger	Mini Bell Peppers Stuffed with Hummus
Day 26	Baked Apple & Oatmeal Cups	Quinoa & Roasted Red Pepper Stuffed Peppers	Stuffed Bell Peppers with Quinoa & Ground Turkey	Roasted Pumpkin Seeds with Sea Salt & Cinnamon
Day 27	Cinnamon-Spiced Chia & Flaxseed Pudding	Grilled Shrimp & Avocado Salad with Cilantro Dressing	Creamy Avocado & Chicken Zoodle Bowl	Sugar-Free Peanut Butter Protein Bars
Day 28	Creamy Peanut Butter & Chia Toast	Quinoa & Roasted Red Pepper Stuffed Peppers	Beef & Mushroom Stir-Fry with Tamari Sauce	Almond Flour Cheddar Crackers
Day 29	Chia & Hemp Seed Protein Smoothie	Balsamic Chicken & Roasted Brussels Sprouts	Cabbage Stir-Fry with Ground Turkey & Ginger	Sautéed Mushrooms & Spinach on Whole Grain Toast
Day 30	Flaxseed & Almond Butter Breakfast Bars	Mediterranean Chickpea & Cucumber Wrap with Tahini Sauce	Stuffed Bell Peppers with Quinoa & Ground Turkey	Baked Zucchini Chips with Parmesan

Tips for Meal Prep and Grocery Shopping on a Budget

Eating well with diabetes doesn't have to mean spending a fortune or spending hours in the kitchen. A strategic approach to meal prep and grocery shopping can make healthy eating more affordable, efficient, and stress-free. The key is to plan ahead, choose nutrient-dense ingredients that won't break the bank, and minimize waste while maximizing variety.

The grocery store can be a minefield of hidden sugars, misleading marketing, and overpriced "health" foods that aren't much better than their processed counterparts. Walking in without a plan often leads to impulse buys, wasted money, and meals that don't align with blood sugar goals. A well-prepared shopping list ensures that every item has a purpose. Structuring meals around whole, unprocessed ingredients makes it easier to stick to a budget while ensuring the body gets the nutrients it needs.

Protein is often the most expensive part of a grocery bill, but it doesn't have to be. Lean cuts of chicken, turkey, and fish can be bought in bulk, portioned out, and frozen for later use. Canned tuna, salmon, and sardines provide high-quality protein and omega-3s at a fraction of the cost of fresh seafood. Eggs are another budget-friendly powerhouse, offering a perfect balance of protein and healthy fats. Plant-based proteins like lentils, black beans, and chickpeas not only cost pennies per serving but also deliver fiber, which helps keep blood sugar stable.

Vegetables don't have to be expensive either. Frozen produce is often just as nutritious as fresh and lasts longer, reducing waste. Buying seasonal produce also cuts costs while ensuring maximum flavor and nutrient content. Root vegetables like carrots and sweet potatoes, leafy greens like spinach and kale, and cruciferous options like broccoli and Brussels sprouts offer a range of vitamins, minerals, and antioxidants without the premium price tag.

Carbohydrates require careful selection. Whole grains like brown rice, quinoa, and oats provide steady energy without causing dramatic blood sugar spikes. Avoiding packaged breads and cereals that claim to be "healthy" but are loaded with refined sugars and preservatives is crucial. Reading labels closely helps separate truly beneficial options from marketing gimmicks.

Meal prep saves both time and money while making healthy eating more convenient. Cooking large batches of soups, stews, and casseroles allows for easy portioning and freezing, ensuring there's always a balanced meal ready to go. Preparing staple ingredients in advance—grilled chicken, roasted vegetables, cooked quinoa—means assembling a quick meal takes minutes instead of hours. Having a go-to list of simple, repeatable meals prevents decision fatigue and eliminates the temptation to grab something unhealthy out of convenience.

A structured approach to grocery shopping and meal prep turns healthy eating into a sustainable habit rather than a daily challenge. By selecting cost-effective, nutrient-dense ingredients and prepping meals ahead of time, it becomes easier to maintain stable blood sugar, avoid food waste, and keep both health and budget on track.

How to Create a Balanced Plate for Blood Sugar Control

Eating with diabetes isn't about depriving yourself—it's about understanding how to build meals that support stable blood sugar while still being satisfying and enjoyable. A well-balanced plate is the foundation of this approach, acting as a roadmap for portions, nutrient distribution, and blood sugar regulation. Every meal should include the right combination of protein, fiber-rich carbohydrates, and healthy fats to create a steady release of glucose into the bloodstream rather than a sudden spike.

The structure of the plate matters. Half of it should be filled with non-starchy vegetables, which provide vitamins, minerals, and fiber without causing blood sugar to rise rapidly. Options like spinach, zucchini, bell peppers, cauliflower, and asparagus add bulk to meals while keeping calories in check. Their fiber slows digestion, helping prevent the rapid absorption of glucose that can lead to blood sugar swings.

A quarter of the plate should contain lean protein. Protein is essential for preserving muscle mass, especially in older adults, and plays a major role in stabilizing blood sugar by slowing down the breakdown of carbohydrates. Choices like grilled chicken, turkey, fish, tofu, and eggs provide essential amino acids without excessive saturated fats. Fatty fish like salmon or sardines offer the added benefit of omega-3 fatty acids, which help reduce inflammation and support heart health.

The remaining quarter should include a controlled portion of carbohydrates. While carbohydrates often get a bad reputation in diabetes management, the key is selecting the right type and amount. Whole grains, legumes, and fiber-rich starchy vegetables like quinoa, lentils, sweet potatoes, and barley offer sustained energy without causing dramatic glucose spikes. These options digest more slowly than refined grains, preventing the rollercoaster of high and low blood sugar that comes with processed foods.

Healthy fats round out the meal, helping with satiety and absorption of fat-soluble vitamins. Avocados, olive oil, nuts, and seeds provide beneficial monounsaturated and polyunsaturated fats that support brain function, hormone balance, and heart health. Fat also helps regulate the release of glucose, working in tandem with fiber and protein to create a slow, even rise in blood sugar rather than a sharp increase.

Portion control plays a critical role. Even the healthiest meal can lead to blood sugar imbalances if portion sizes are excessive. Measuring out servings, using smaller plates, and being mindful of hunger cues can prevent overeating while ensuring the body gets exactly what it needs. Over time, consistently eating in balanced proportions helps improve insulin sensitivity, maintain energy levels, and reduce the risk of complications.

A structured eating plan removes uncertainty and makes healthy choices second nature. Knowing how to balance meals, shop wisely, and prepare food efficiently sets the stage for long-term success. Small, intentional habits add up, leading to better blood sugar control, increased energy, and a way of eating that feels both natural and sustainable.

Chapter 2: Energizing Breakfasts to Start Your Day Right

CINNAMON-SPICED CHIA & FLAXSEED PUDDING

P.T.: 5 minutes (preparation), 0 minutes (cooking)

Ingr.:
- 2 tbsp chia seeds
- 1 tbsp ground flaxseed
- 1 cup unsweetened almond milk
- ½ tsp ground cinnamon
- ½ tsp vanilla extract
- 1 tsp monk fruit sweetener

Serv.: 2

Method of Cooking: No-cook, refrigeration

Procedure:

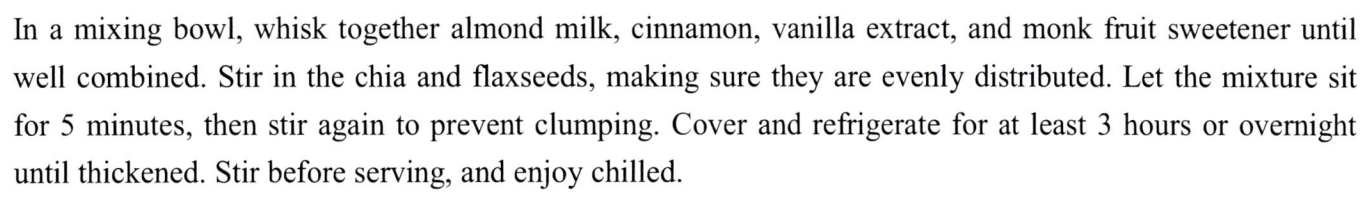

In a mixing bowl, whisk together almond milk, cinnamon, vanilla extract, and monk fruit sweetener until well combined. Stir in the chia and flaxseeds, making sure they are evenly distributed. Let the mixture sit for 5 minutes, then stir again to prevent clumping. Cover and refrigerate for at least 3 hours or overnight until thickened. Stir before serving, and enjoy chilled.

N.V.: (per serving) Cal. 120 | Fat 7g | Carb. 9g | Prot. 4g

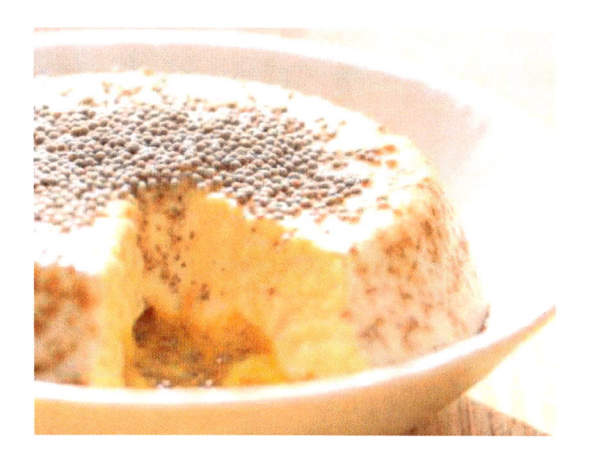

SAVORY COTTAGE CHEESE & AVOCADO TOAST ON SPROUTED GRAIN BREAD

P.T.: 5 minutes (preparation), 0 minutes (cooking)

Ingr.:
- 2 slices sprouted grain bread
- ½ cup cottage cheese
- ½ small avocado, mashed
- ¼ tsp smoked paprika
- 1 tsp lemon juice
- Salt & black pepper to taste

Serv.: 2

Method of Cooking: No-cook

Procedure:

Toast the sprouted grain bread to desired crispiness. In a small bowl, mix mashed avocado with lemon juice, smoked paprika, salt, and black pepper. Spread cottage cheese evenly over each slice of toast, then top with the avocado mixture. Serve immediately.

N.V.: (per serving) Cal. 180 | Fat 7g | Carb. 18g | Prot. 10g

PUMPKIN PIE OATMEAL WITH WALNUTS & GREEK YOGURT

P.T.: 5 minutes (preparation), 5 minutes (cooking)

Ingr.:
- ½ cup rolled oats
- 1 cup unsweetened almond milk
- 2 tbsp pumpkin purée
- ¼ tsp pumpkin spice
- 1 tbsp chopped walnuts
- ¼ cup plain Greek yogurt

Serv.: 2

Method of Cooking: Stovetop

Procedure:

In a saucepan, bring almond milk to a simmer over medium heat. Stir in oats and cook for 3-5 minutes, stirring occasionally. Add pumpkin purée and pumpkin spice, mixing well until creamy. Remove from heat and divide into bowls. Top each serving with chopped walnuts and a spoonful of Greek yogurt before serving.

N.V.: (per serving) Cal. 210 | Fat 7g | Carb. 28g | Prot. 9g

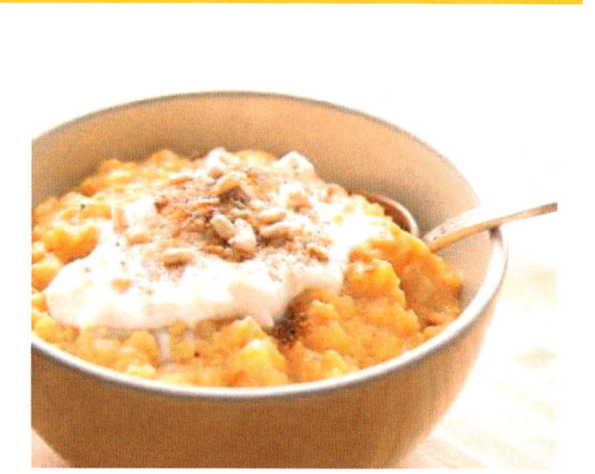

EGG & SPINACH BREAKFAST MUFFINS

P.T.: 5 minutes (preparation), 15 minutes (cooking)

Ingr.:
- 4 large eggs
- ½ cup fresh spinach, chopped
- ¼ cup shredded cheddar cheese
- ¼ tsp garlic powder
- ¼ tsp salt
- ¼ tsp black pepper

Serv.: 2

Method of Cooking: Baking

Procedure:

Preheat the oven to 350°F and lightly grease a muffin tin. In a bowl, whisk eggs, garlic powder, salt, and black pepper. Stir in spinach and cheese. Pour the mixture into muffin cups, filling each about three-quarters full. Bake for 15 minutes or until eggs are set. Let cool slightly before serving.

N.V.: (per serving) Cal. 170 | Fat 11g | Carb. 3g | Prot. 14g

BLUEBERRY ALMOND FLOUR PANCAKES

P.T.: 5 minutes (preparation), 10 minutes (cooking)

Ingr.:
- ½ cup almond flour
- 1 large egg
- ¼ cup unsweetened almond milk
- ½ tsp baking powder
- ¼ cup fresh blueberries
- ½ tsp vanilla extract

Serv.: 2

Method of Cooking: Stovetop

Procedure:

In a bowl, whisk egg, almond milk, and vanilla extract until smooth. Stir in almond flour and baking powder until a batter forms. Fold in blueberries. Heat a non-stick skillet over medium heat and lightly grease. Pour small amounts of batter onto the skillet, cooking for 2-3 minutes per side until golden brown. Serve warm.

N.V.: (per serving) Cal. 190 | Fat 13g | Carb. 9g | Prot. 7g

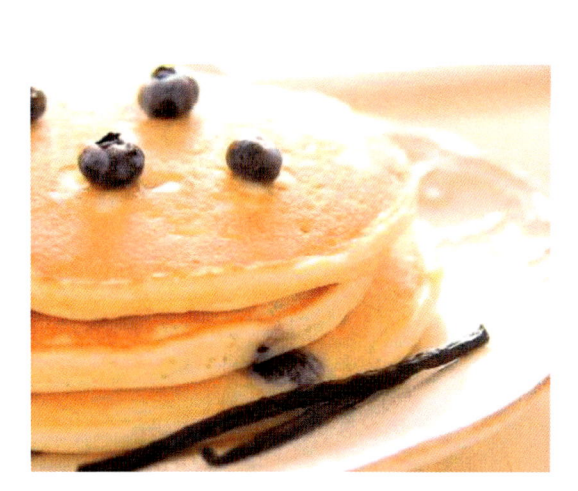

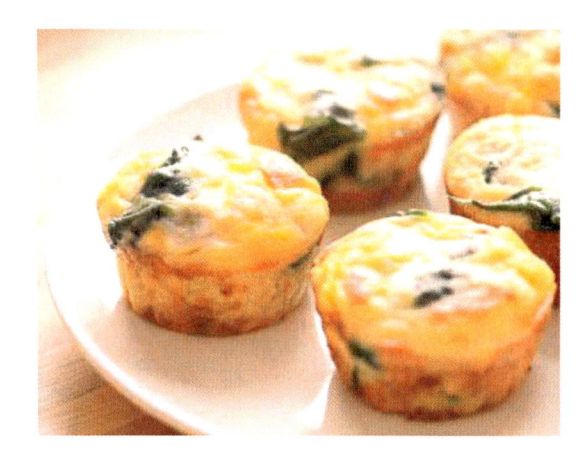

ZUCCHINI & CHEDDAR OMELET ROLL-UPS

P.T.: 5 minutes (preparation), 5 minutes (cooking)

Ingr.:
- 2 large eggs
- ¼ cup shredded cheddar cheese
- ¼ cup zucchini, grated
- 1 tbsp chopped chives
- ¼ tsp salt
- ¼ tsp black pepper

Serv.: 2

Method of Cooking: Stovetop

Procedure:

In a bowl, whisk eggs, salt, and black pepper. Heat a non-stick skillet over medium heat and pour the mixture in, tilting the pan for an even layer. Sprinkle grated zucchini and cheddar cheese evenly on top. Cook until set, about 3 minutes. Roll the omelet into a log, slice in half, and garnish with chives before serving.

N.V.: (per serving) Cal. 160 | Fat 11g | Carb. 3g | Prot. 12g

CHIA & HEMP SEED PROTEIN SMOOTHIE

P.T.: 5 minutes (preparation), 0 minutes (cooking)

Ingr.:
- 1 cup unsweetened almond milk
- 1 tbsp chia seeds
- 1 tbsp hemp seeds
- ¼ cup frozen mixed berries
- ½ tsp vanilla extract
- 1 tsp monk fruit sweetener

Serv.: 2

Method of Cooking: Blending

Procedure:

Combine all ingredients in a blender and blend on high speed until smooth. Pour into glasses and serve immediately.

N.V.: (per serving) Cal. 150 | Fat 8g | Carb. 10g | Prot. 6g

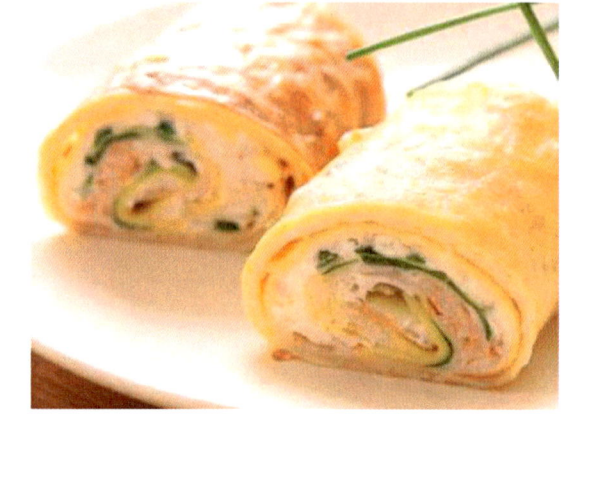

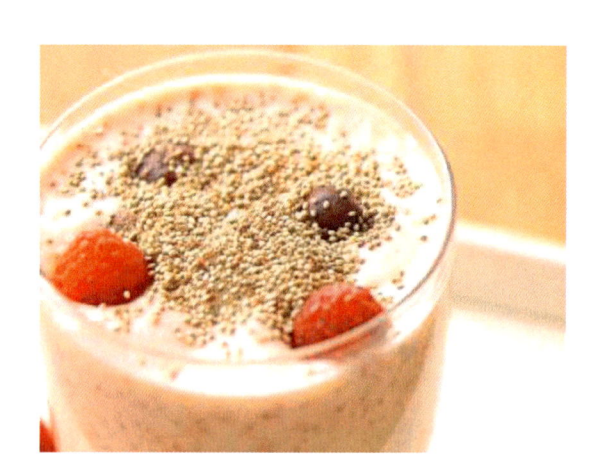

BAKED APPLE & OATMEAL CUPS

P.T.: 5 minutes (preparation), 20 minutes (cooking)

Ingr.:
- ½ cup rolled oats
- 1 small apple, diced
- ½ cup unsweetened almond milk
- ½ tsp cinnamon
- 1 egg
- 1 tsp baking powder

Serv.: 2

Method of Cooking: Baking

Procedure:

Preheat oven to 350°F and grease a muffin tin. In a bowl, mix oats, apple, cinnamon, baking powder, almond milk, and egg until combined. Pour into muffin cups and bake for 20 minutes. Let cool slightly before serving.

N.V.: (per serving) Cal. 180 | Fat 5g | Carb. 25g | Prot. 6g

AVOCADO & SMOKED SALMON SCRAMBLE

P.T.: 5 minutes (preparation), 5 minutes (cooking)

Ingr.:
- 2 large eggs
- ¼ small avocado, diced
- 1 oz smoked salmon, chopped
- ¼ tsp black pepper
- 1 tsp olive oil
- 1 tbsp chopped dill

Serv.: 2

Method of Cooking: Stovetop

Procedure:

In a bowl, whisk eggs and black pepper. Heat olive oil in a skillet over medium heat, then add eggs, stirring gently. When eggs begin to set, fold in avocado and smoked salmon. Cook for another minute until eggs are just set. Garnish with dill and serve immediately.

N.V.: (per serving) Cal. 200 | Fat 14g | Carb. 3g | Prot. 16g

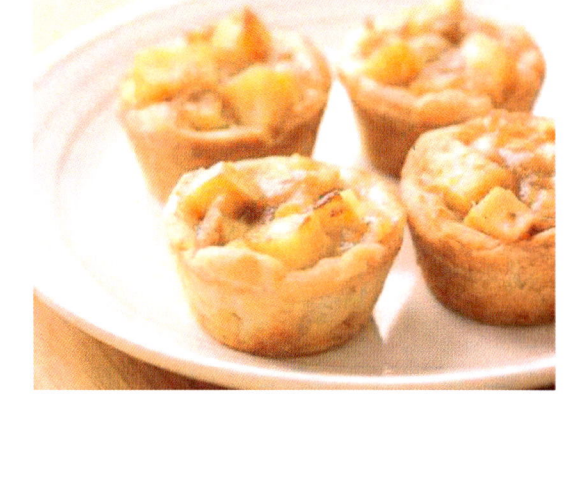

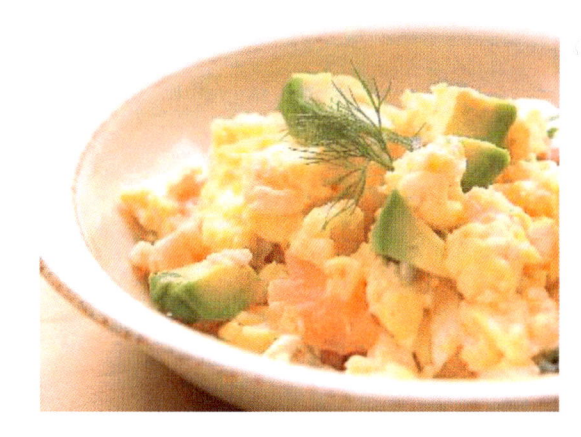

COCONUT & PECAN OVERNIGHT OATS

P.T.: 5 minutes (preparation), 0 minutes (cooking)

Ingr.:
- ½ cup rolled oats
- 1 cup unsweetened coconut milk
- 1 tbsp shredded unsweetened coconut
- 1 tbsp chopped pecans
- ½ tsp cinnamon
- 1 tsp monk fruit sweetener

Serv.: 2

Method of Cooking: No-cook, refrigeration

Procedure:

In a jar or bowl, mix oats, coconut milk, shredded coconut, cinnamon, and monk fruit sweetener. Stir well and refrigerate overnight. Before serving, sprinkle with chopped pecans. Serve chilled.

N.V.: (per serving) Cal. 210 | Fat 10g | Carb. 26g | Prot. 5g

CAULIFLOWER & CHEESE BREAKFAST HASH

P.T.: 5 minutes (preparation), 10 minutes (cooking)

Ingr.:
- 1 cup riced cauliflower
- ½ cup shredded cheddar cheese
- ½ small onion, diced
- 1 tbsp olive oil
- ¼ tsp smoked paprika
- ¼ tsp black pepper

Serv.: 2

Method of Cooking: Stovetop

Procedure:

Heat olive oil in a skillet over medium heat. Sauté diced onion until translucent, then add riced cauliflower, smoked paprika, and black pepper. Cook for 5 minutes, stirring occasionally. Sprinkle cheddar cheese on top, cover, and cook for another 3 minutes until cheese melts. Serve warm.

N.V.: (per serving) Cal. 180 | Fat 12g | Carb. 8g | Prot. 10g

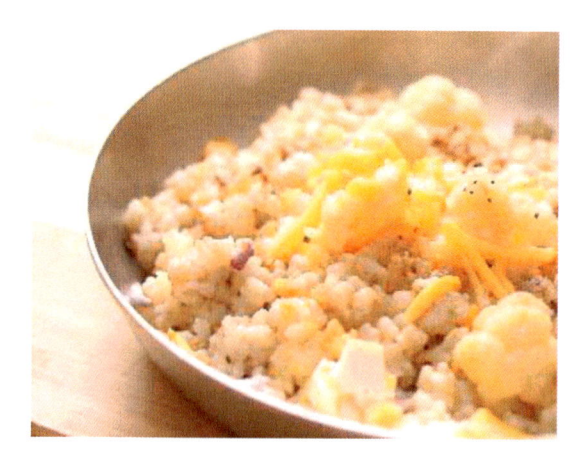

FLAXSEED & ALMOND BUTTER BREAKFAST BARS

P.T.: 5 minutes (preparation), 15 minutes (cooking)

Ingr.:
- ½ cup ground flaxseeds
- ¼ cup almond butter
- ¼ cup unsweetened applesauce
- 1 tbsp chia seeds
- ½ tsp vanilla extract
- 1 tsp cinnamon

Serv.: 2

Method of Cooking: Baking

Procedure:

Preheat oven to 350°F and line a baking sheet with parchment paper. In a bowl, mix all ingredients until a thick dough forms. Press mixture into a small square, about ½-inch thick. Bake for 15 minutes until set. Let cool before slicing into bars.

N.V.: (per serving) Cal. 190 | Fat 13g | Carb. 9g | Prot. 6g

MUSHROOM & FETA BREAKFAST WRAP

P.T.: 5 minutes (preparation), 5 minutes (cooking)

Ingr.:
- 2 large eggs
- ¼ cup sliced mushrooms
- ¼ cup crumbled feta cheese
- 1 low-carb whole wheat tortilla
- 1 tsp olive oil
- ¼ tsp black pepper

Serv.: 2

Method of Cooking: Stovetop

Procedure:

Heat olive oil in a skillet over medium heat. Sauté mushrooms until soft, then remove from skillet. In the same skillet, scramble eggs with black pepper. Place scrambled eggs, mushrooms, and feta cheese in the center of a tortilla, then roll into a wrap. Serve warm.

N.V.: (per serving) Cal. 220 | Fat 12g | Carb. 14g | Prot. 14g

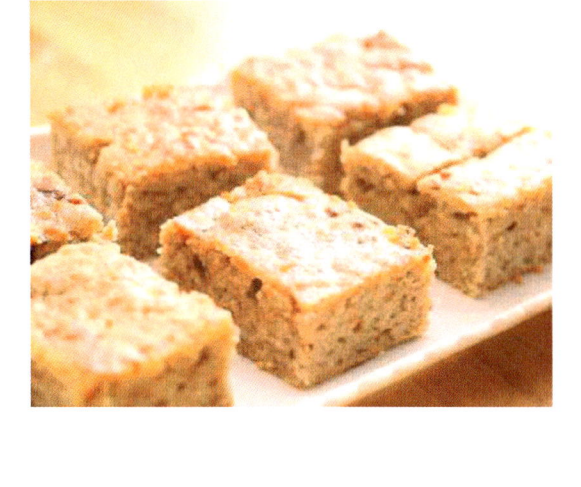

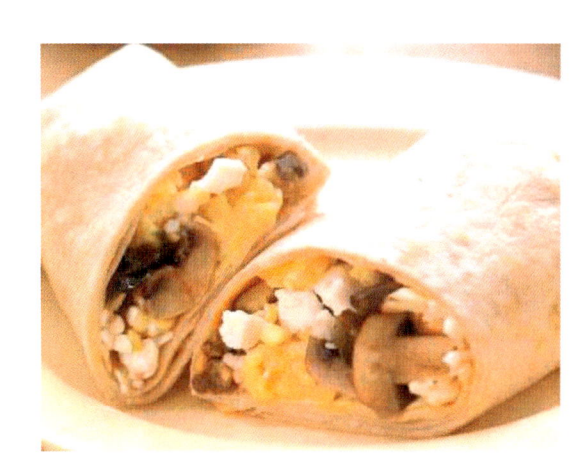

VANILLA RICOTTA & BERRY PARFAIT

P.T.: 5 minutes (preparation), 0 minutes (cooking)

Ingr.:
- ½ cup ricotta cheese
- ¼ cup mixed berries (blueberries, raspberries, strawberries)
- ½ tsp vanilla extract
- 1 tsp chia seeds
- 1 tsp monk fruit sweetener
- 1 tbsp crushed walnuts

Serv.: 2

Method of Cooking: No-cook

Procedure:

In a bowl, mix ricotta cheese, vanilla extract, and monk fruit sweetener until smooth. Layer ricotta mixture with berries in serving cups. Sprinkle chia seeds and walnuts on top. Serve immediately.

N.V.: (per serving) Cal. 180 | Fat 10g | Carb. 9g | Prot. 12g

SAVORY SWEET POTATO & EGG BOWL

P.T.: 5 minutes (preparation), 10 minutes (cooking)

Ingr.:
- ½ cup diced sweet potatoes
- 2 large eggs
- 1 tbsp olive oil
- ¼ tsp smoked paprika
- ¼ tsp garlic powder
- Salt & black pepper to taste

Serv.: 2

Method of Cooking: Stovetop

Procedure:

Heat olive oil in a skillet over medium heat. Sauté diced sweet potatoes with smoked paprika and garlic powder for 8 minutes, stirring occasionally. In the same skillet, scramble eggs until just set. Season with salt and black pepper. Serve eggs over sweet potatoes.

N.V.: (per serving) Cal. 210 | Fat 11g | Carb. 18g | Prot. 10g

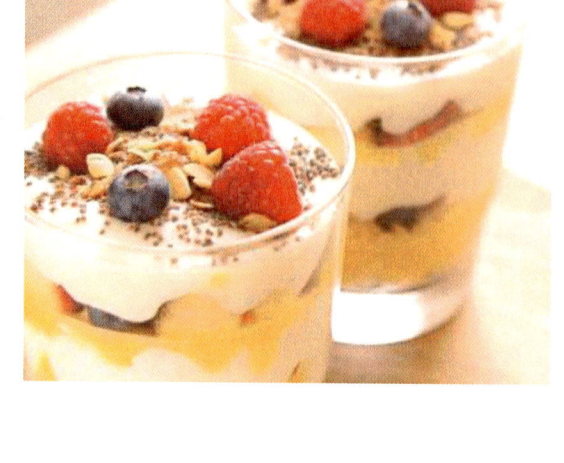

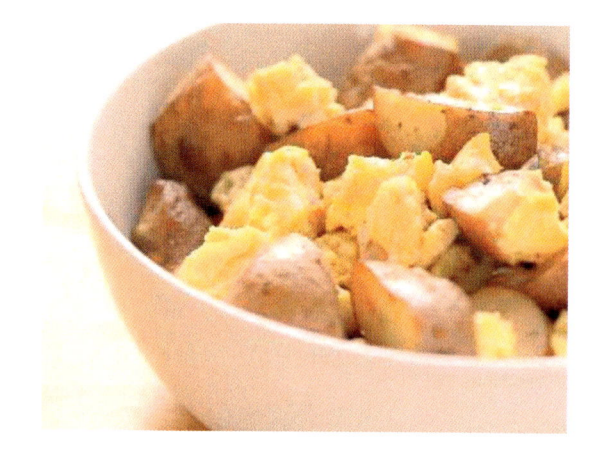

GREEN POWER BREAKFAST SCRAMBLE (KALE, EGGS & TURKEY SAUSAGE)

P.T.: 5 minutes (preparation), 10 minutes (cooking)

Ingr.:
- 2 large eggs
- ½ cup chopped kale
- 1 turkey sausage, crumbled
- 1 tbsp olive oil
- ¼ tsp red pepper flakes
- ¼ tsp black pepper

Serv.: 2

Method of Cooking: Stovetop

Procedure:

Heat olive oil in a skillet over medium heat. Cook turkey sausage until browned. Add kale and red pepper flakes, stirring until wilted. Crack eggs directly into the skillet and scramble with a spatula. Cook until eggs are set. Serve warm.

N.V.: (per serving) Cal. 230 | Fat 14g | Carb. 6g | Prot. 18g

SUGAR-FREE BANANA WALNUT MUFFINS

P.T.: 5 minutes (preparation), 15 minutes (cooking)

Ingr.:
- ½ cup almond flour
- 1 ripe banana, mashed
- 1 large egg
- 1 tsp baking powder
- 1 tbsp chopped walnuts
- ½ tsp cinnamon

Serv.: 2

Method of Cooking: Baking

Procedure:

Preheat oven to 350°F. In a bowl, mix mashed banana, egg, almond flour, baking powder, and cinnamon until combined. Fold in walnuts. Divide batter into muffin cups and bake for 15 minutes until golden. Let cool before serving.

N.V.: (per serving) Cal. 180 | Fat 10g | Carb. 15g | Prot. 7g

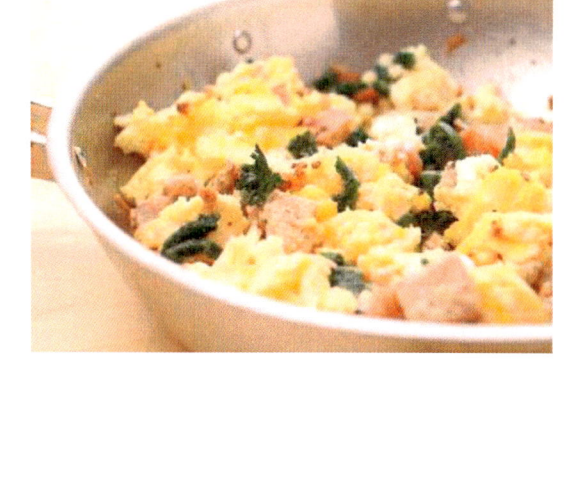

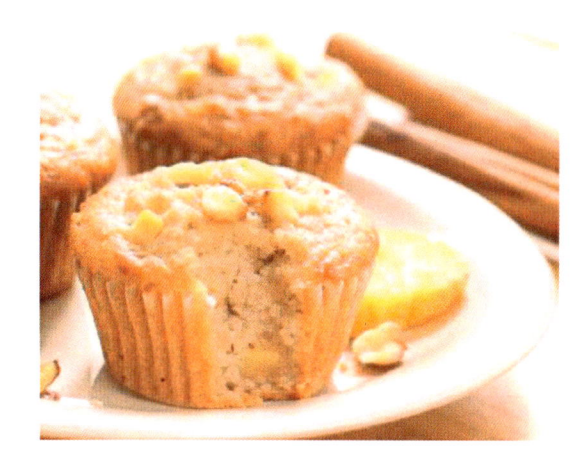

SPICED QUINOA BREAKFAST BOWL WITH ALMONDS & COCONUT MILK

P.T.: 5 minutes (preparation), 10 minutes (cooking)

Ingr.:
- ½ cup cooked quinoa
- ½ cup unsweetened coconut milk
- 1 tbsp sliced almonds
- ½ tsp cinnamon
- 1 tsp monk fruit sweetener
- ½ tsp vanilla extract

Serv.: 2

Method of Cooking: Stovetop

Procedure:

In a saucepan over medium heat, warm quinoa with coconut milk, cinnamon, monk fruit sweetener, and vanilla extract. Stir well and cook for 5 minutes until heated through. Divide into bowls and top with sliced almonds.

N.V.: (per serving) Cal. 190 | Fat 9g | Carb. 20g | Prot. 6g

CREAMY PEANUT BUTTER & CHIA TOAST ON WHOLE GRAIN RYE

P.T.: 5 minutes (preparation), 0 minutes (cooking)

Ingr.:
- 2 slices whole grain rye bread
- 2 tbsp natural peanut butter
- 1 tsp chia seeds
- ½ tsp cinnamon
- ½ tsp vanilla extract
- 1 tsp monk fruit sweetener

Serv.: 2

Method of Cooking: No-cook

Procedure:

Spread peanut butter evenly over rye bread. Sprinkle with chia seeds, cinnamon, and monk fruit sweetener. Serve immediately.

N.V.: (per serving) Cal. 200 | Fat 12g | Carb. 15g | Prot. 8g

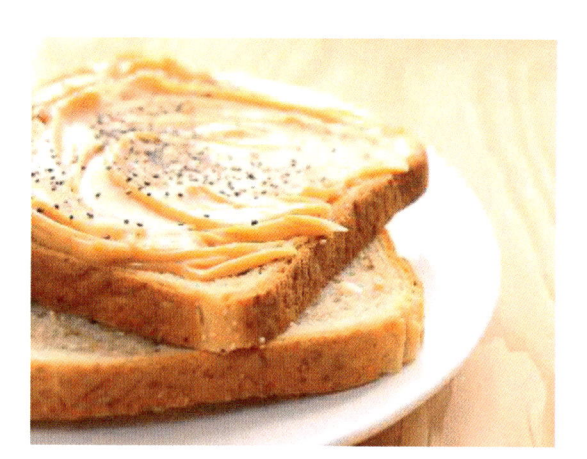

GOLDEN TURMERIC SMOOTHIE WITH GREEK YOGURT & ALMOND MILK

P.T.: 5 minutes (preparation), 0 minutes (cooking)

Ingr.:
- ½ cup plain Greek yogurt
- ½ cup unsweetened almond milk
- ½ tsp ground turmeric
- ¼ tsp ground ginger
- 1 tsp monk fruit sweetener
- ½ tsp vanilla extract

Serv.: 2

Method of Cooking: Blending

Procedure:

Combine Greek yogurt, almond milk, turmeric, ginger, monk fruit sweetener, and vanilla extract in a blender. Blend on high speed until smooth and creamy. Pour into glasses and serve immediately.

N.V.: (per serving) Cal. 120 | Fat 4g | Carb. 10g | Prot. 10g

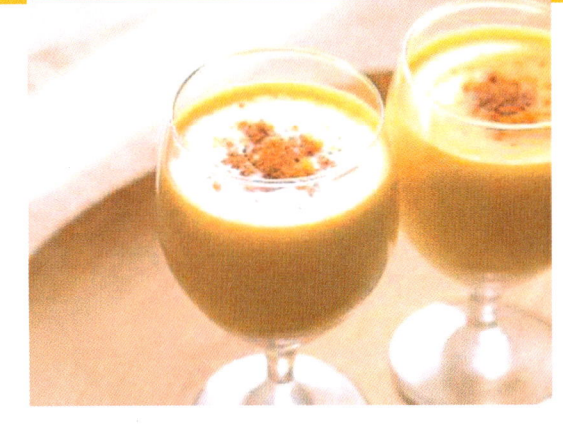

Chapter 3: Flavorful Lunches for Balanced Blood Sugar

GRILLED LEMON HERB CHICKEN WITH QUINOA & ROASTED VEGGIES

P.T.: 10 minutes (preparation), 20 minutes (cooking)

Ingr.:
- 2 small boneless, skinless chicken breasts
- ½ cup quinoa, rinsed
- 1 cup broccoli florets
- ½ red bell pepper, sliced
- 1 tbsp olive oil
- Juice of ½ lemon

Serv.: 2

Method of Cooking: Grilling, roasting, stovetop

Procedure:

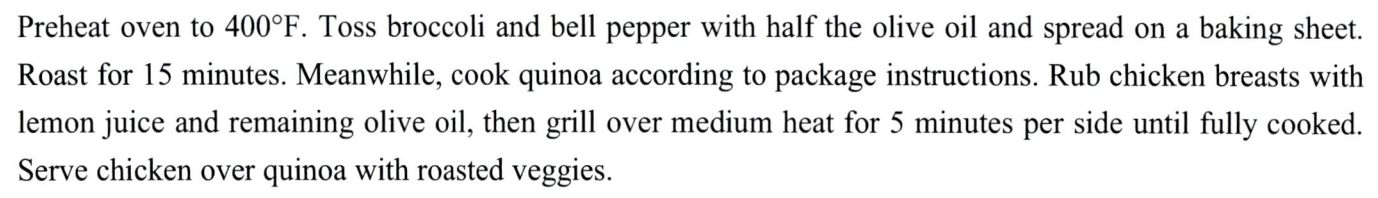

Preheat oven to 400°F. Toss broccoli and bell pepper with half the olive oil and spread on a baking sheet. Roast for 15 minutes. Meanwhile, cook quinoa according to package instructions. Rub chicken breasts with lemon juice and remaining olive oil, then grill over medium heat for 5 minutes per side until fully cooked. Serve chicken over quinoa with roasted veggies.

N.V.: (per serving) Cal. 320 | Fat 10g | Carb. 28g | Prot. 30g

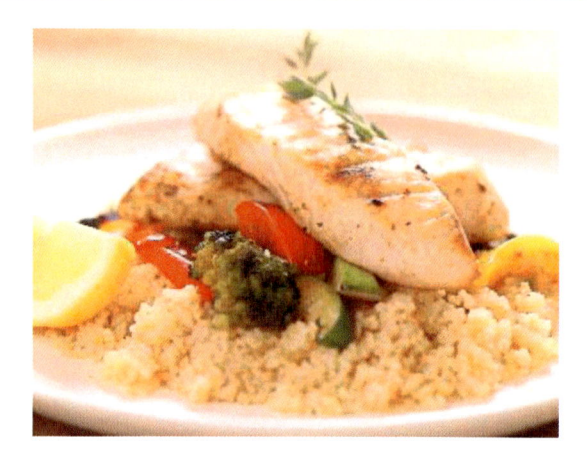

SPINACH & FETA STUFFED PORTOBELLO MUSHROOMS

P.T.: 10 minutes (preparation), 15 minutes (cooking)

Ingr.:
- 2 large Portobello mushrooms
- 1 cup fresh spinach, chopped
- ¼ cup crumbled feta cheese
- 1 tbsp olive oil
- ¼ tsp garlic powder
- ¼ tsp black pepper

Serv.: 2

Method of Cooking: Baking

Procedure:

Preheat oven to 375°F. Remove stems from mushrooms and brush with olive oil. In a skillet, sauté spinach until wilted, then mix with feta, garlic powder, and black pepper. Stuff mixture into mushrooms and bake for 15 minutes until tender. Serve warm.

N.V.: (per serving) Cal. 190 | Fat 12g | Carb. 10g | Prot. 12g

ZESTY BLACK BEAN & AVOCADO SALAD WITH LIME DRESSING

P.T.: 5 minutes (preparation), 0 minutes (cooking)

Ingr.:
- ½ cup black beans, drained and rinsed
- ½ avocado, diced
- ¼ cup cherry tomatoes, halved
- 1 tbsp fresh lime juice
- 1 tsp olive oil
- ¼ tsp cumin

Serv.: 2

Method of Cooking: No-cook

Procedure:

In a bowl, mix black beans, avocado, and cherry tomatoes. Drizzle with lime juice, olive oil, and sprinkle with cumin. Toss gently to combine. Serve immediately.

N.V.: (per serving) Cal. 210 | Fat 10g | Carb. 22g | Prot. 7g

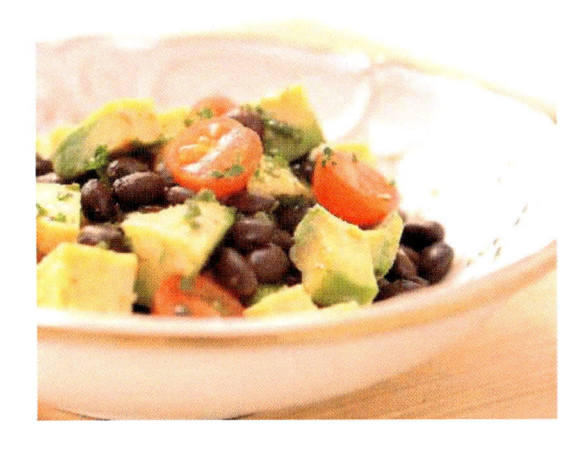

CAULIFLOWER RICE STIR-FRY WITH TOFU & SESAME GINGER SAUCE

P.T.: 10 minutes (preparation), 10 minutes (cooking)

Ingr.:
- 1 cup cauliflower rice
- ½ cup firm tofu, cubed
- 1 tbsp low-sodium soy sauce
- 1 tsp sesame oil
- ½ tsp grated ginger
- ¼ cup shredded carrots

Serv.: 2

Method of Cooking: Stir-frying

Procedure:

Heat sesame oil in a skillet over medium heat. Add tofu and cook until golden brown. Stir in ginger, shredded carrots, and cauliflower rice. Pour in soy sauce and stir-fry for 5 minutes until heated through. Serve warm.

N.V.: (per serving) Cal. 180 | Fat 8g | Carb. 14g | Prot. 12g

MEDITERRANEAN CHICKPEA & CUCUMBER WRAP WITH TAHINI SAUCE

P.T.: 5 minutes (preparation), 0 minutes (cooking)

Ingr.:
- ½ cup chickpeas, drained and rinsed
- ½ small cucumber, diced
- 1 tbsp tahini
- 1 tsp lemon juice
- 1 low-carb whole wheat tortilla
- ¼ tsp ground cumin

Serv.: 2

Method of Cooking: No-cook

Procedure:

Mash chickpeas lightly in a bowl. Add cucumber, tahini, lemon juice, and cumin, stirring well. Spread mixture onto a whole wheat tortilla, roll tightly, and slice in half. Serve chilled.

N.V.: (per serving) Cal. 230 | Fat 9g | Carb. 28g | Prot. 9g

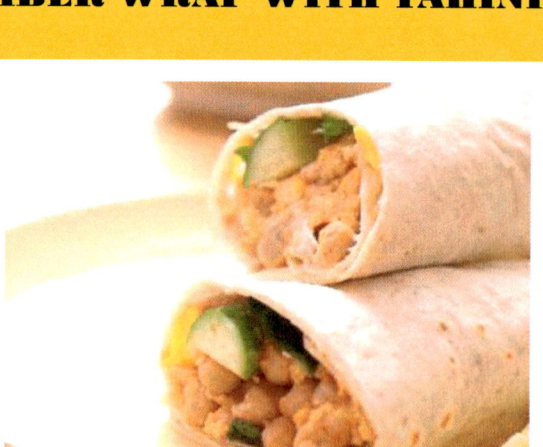

BAKED SALMON WITH GARLIC BUTTER & ASPARAGUS

P.T.: 5 minutes (preparation), 15 minutes (cooking)

Ingr.:
- 2 small salmon fillets
- 1 tbsp butter, melted
- ½ tsp garlic powder
- ½ tsp lemon zest
- ½ cup asparagus spears
- ¼ tsp salt

Serv.: 2

Method of Cooking: Baking

Procedure:

Preheat oven to 375°F. Place salmon fillets and asparagus on a baking sheet. Drizzle with melted butter, sprinkle with garlic powder, lemon zest, and salt. Bake for 15 minutes until salmon flakes easily. Serve warm.

N.V.: (per serving) Cal. 320 | Fat 18g | Carb. 6g | Prot. 30g

SPICY TURKEY & ZUCCHINI MEATBALLS WITH TOMATO BASIL SAUCE

P.T.: 10 minutes (preparation), 20 minutes (cooking)

Ingr.:
- ½ lb ground turkey
- ½ cup grated zucchini
- ¼ tsp red pepper flakes
- ½ cup crushed tomatoes
- ½ tsp dried basil
- 1 tbsp olive oil

Serv.: 2

Method of Cooking: Stovetop

Procedure:

In a bowl, mix ground turkey, grated zucchini, and red pepper flakes. Shape into small meatballs. Heat olive oil in a pan and brown meatballs on all sides. Pour in crushed tomatoes and basil, then simmer for 10 minutes. Serve warm.

N.V.: (per serving) Cal. 280 | Fat 14g | Carb. 10g | Prot. 30g

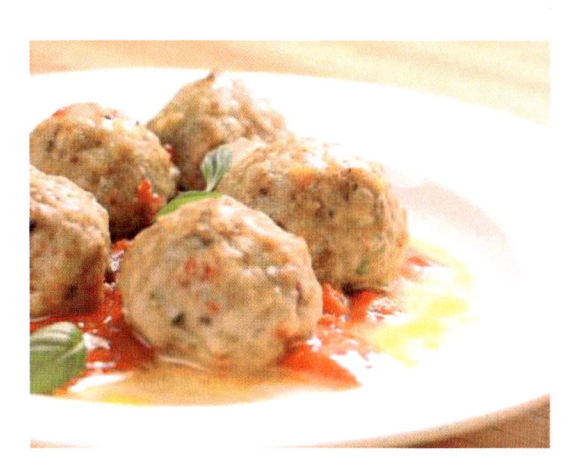

ROASTED SWEET POTATO & KALE SALAD WITH WALNUTS & FETA

P.T.: 10 minutes (preparation), 20 minutes (cooking)

Ingr.:
- ½ cup diced sweet potatoes
- 1 cup chopped kale
- 1 tbsp chopped walnuts
- ¼ cup crumbled feta cheese
- 1 tbsp olive oil
- ¼ tsp black pepper

Serv.: 2

Method of Cooking: Roasting

Procedure:

Preheat oven to 400°F. Toss sweet potatoes with olive oil and roast for 20 minutes until tender. Massage kale with a drizzle of olive oil. Toss roasted sweet potatoes with kale, walnuts, and feta. Serve warm.

N.V.: (per serving) Cal. 250 | Fat 14g | Carb. 22g | Prot. 8g

TUNA & WHITE BEAN SALAD WITH OLIVE OIL & LEMON

P.T.: 5 minutes (preparation), 0 minutes (cooking)

Ingr.:
- 1 can tuna in water, drained
- ½ cup white beans, drained and rinsed
- 1 tbsp olive oil
- 1 tsp lemon juice
- ¼ tsp black pepper
- 1 tbsp chopped parsley

Serv.: 2

Method of Cooking: No-cook

Procedure:

In a bowl, mix tuna, white beans, olive oil, lemon juice, black pepper, and parsley until well combined. Serve chilled.

N.V.: (per serving) Cal. 220 | Fat 10g | Carb. 12g | Prot. 20g

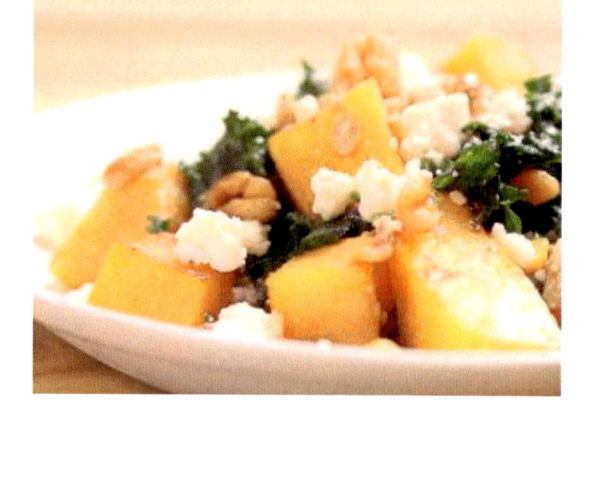

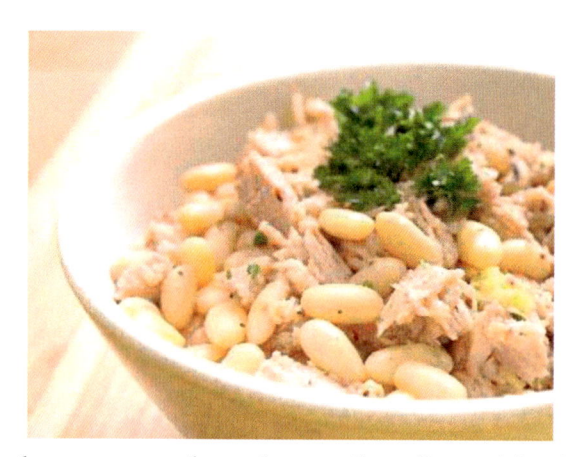

HEARTY LENTIL & SPINACH SOUP WITH TURMERIC

P.T.: 10 minutes (preparation), 20 minutes (cooking)

Ingr.:
- ½ cup dry lentils
- 1 cup fresh spinach, chopped
- ½ tsp ground turmeric
- 2 cups low-sodium vegetable broth
- 1 tsp olive oil
- ¼ tsp black pepper

Serv.: 2

Method of Cooking: Stovetop

Procedure:

Heat olive oil in a pot over medium heat. Add lentils, turmeric, and black pepper, stirring for a minute. Pour in vegetable broth and simmer for 15 minutes. Add spinach and cook for another 5 minutes until wilted. Serve warm.

N.V.: (per serving) Cal. 200 | Fat 4g | Carb. 28g | Prot. 12g

GRILLED SHRIMP & AVOCADO SALAD WITH CILANTRO DRESSING

P.T.: 10 minutes (preparation), 5 minutes (cooking)

Ingr.:
- 6 medium shrimp, peeled and deveined
- ½ avocado, diced
- 1 cup mixed greens
- 1 tbsp chopped cilantro
- 1 tbsp olive oil
- 1 tsp lime juice

Serv.: 2

Method of Cooking: Grilling

Procedure:

Heat a grill pan over medium heat and brush with olive oil. Grill shrimp for 2-3 minutes per side until pink and opaque. Toss mixed greens with avocado and grilled shrimp. In a small bowl, whisk lime juice, cilantro, and olive oil to make a dressing. Drizzle over salad and serve immediately.

N.V.: (per serving) Cal. 230 | Fat 14g | Carb. 8g | Prot. 18g

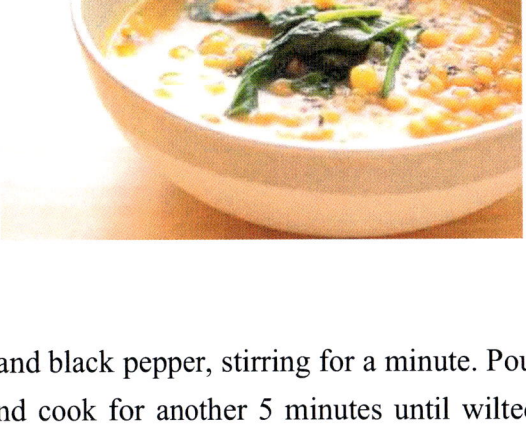

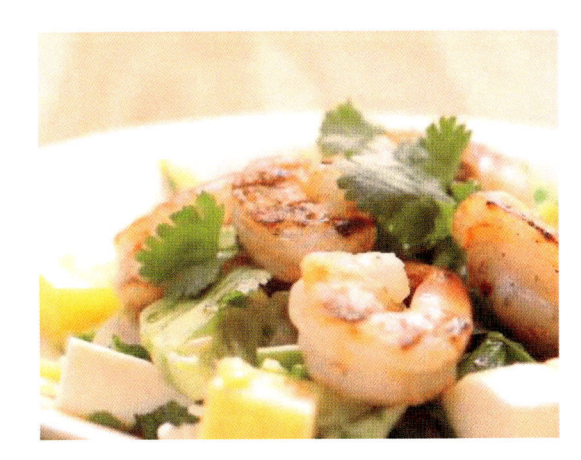

COTTAGE CHEESE & CUCUMBER LETTUCE WRAPS

P.T.: 5 minutes (preparation), 0 minutes (cooking)

Ingr.:
- ½ cup cottage cheese
- ½ small cucumber, diced
- 2 large lettuce leaves
- ¼ tsp black pepper
- ¼ tsp garlic powder
- 1 tsp lemon juice

Serv.: 2

Method of Cooking: No-cook

Procedure:

In a bowl, mix cottage cheese, cucumber, lemon juice, black pepper, and garlic powder. Spoon mixture into lettuce leaves and fold like a wrap. Serve immediately.

N.V.: (per serving) Cal. 150 | Fat 5g | Carb. 6g | Prot. 14g

BALSAMIC CHICKEN & ROASTED BRUSSELS SPROUTS

P.T.: 10 minutes (preparation), 20 minutes (cooking)

Ingr.:
- 2 small boneless chicken breasts
- 1 cup Brussels sprouts, halved
- 1 tbsp balsamic vinegar
- 1 tbsp olive oil
- ¼ tsp salt
- ¼ tsp black pepper

Serv.: 2

Method of Cooking: Roasting

Procedure:

Preheat oven to 400°F. Toss Brussels sprouts with half the olive oil, salt, and black pepper, then spread on a baking sheet. Roast for 15 minutes. Meanwhile, rub chicken with balsamic vinegar and remaining olive oil. Place chicken on the same baking sheet and roast for an additional 10 minutes, or until cooked through. Serve warm.

N.V.: (per serving) Cal. 280 | Fat 12g | Carb. 10g | Prot. 32g

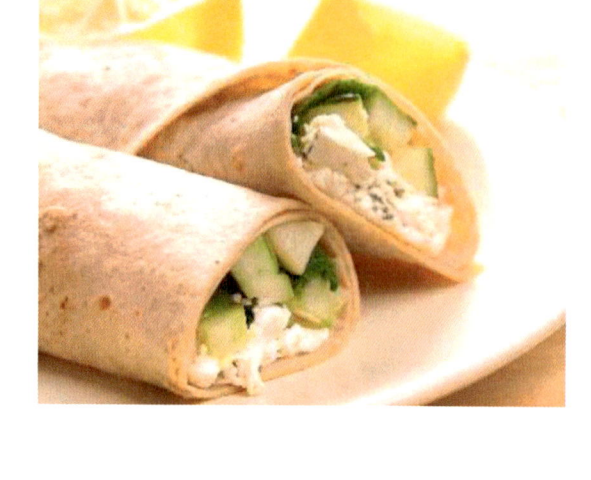

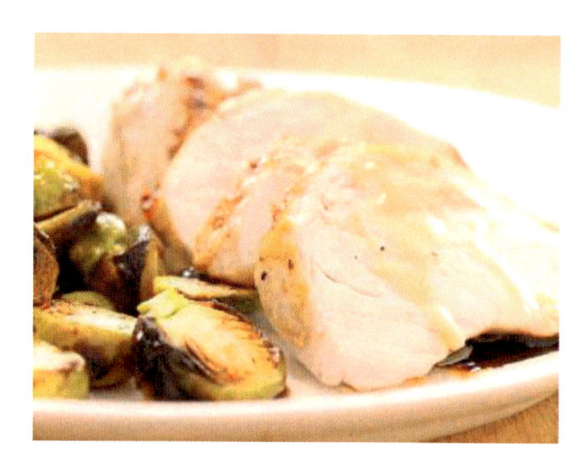

SAUTÉED GARLIC TOFU & BOK CHOY OVER BROWN RICE

P.T.: 10 minutes (preparation), 10 minutes (cooking)

Ingr.:
- ½ cup firm tofu, cubed
- 1 cup chopped bok choy
- ½ cup cooked brown rice
- 1 tsp sesame oil
- ½ tsp minced garlic
- 1 tbsp low-sodium soy sauce

Serv.: 2

Method of Cooking: Stir-frying

Procedure:

Heat sesame oil in a skillet over medium heat. Add tofu and cook until golden brown. Stir in garlic and bok choy, cooking for 3 minutes. Pour in soy sauce and mix well. Serve over brown rice.

N.V.: (per serving) Cal. 220 | Fat 8g | Carb. 22g | Prot. 14g

CREAMY AVOCADO & CHICKEN SALAD ON WHOLE GRAIN TOAST

P.T.: 5 minutes (preparation), 0 minutes (cooking)

Ingr.:
- ½ avocado, mashed
- ½ cup cooked shredded chicken
- 1 tsp lemon juice
- ¼ tsp black pepper
- 2 slices whole grain toast
- 1 tsp olive oil

Serv.: 2

Method of Cooking: No-cook

Procedure:

In a bowl, mix mashed avocado, shredded chicken, lemon juice, and black pepper. Spread onto toasted whole grain bread and drizzle with olive oil. Serve immediately.

N.V.: (per serving) Cal. 250 | Fat 14g | Carb. 18g | Prot. 18g

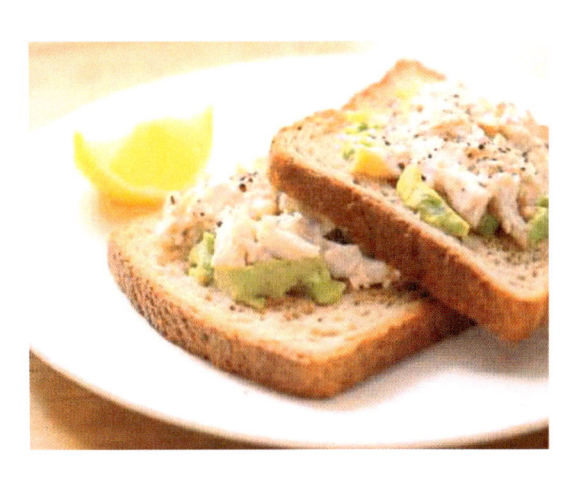

BEEF & BROCCOLI STIR-FRY WITH TAMARI SAUCE

P.T.: 10 minutes (preparation), 10 minutes (cooking)

Ingr.:
- 4 oz lean beef, sliced thin
- 1 cup broccoli florets
- 1 tbsp low-sodium tamari sauce
- 1 tsp sesame oil
- ½ tsp minced ginger
- ¼ tsp black pepper

Serv.: 2

Method of Cooking: Stir-frying

Procedure:

Heat sesame oil in a pan over medium heat. Add beef and cook until browned. Stir in ginger, black pepper, and broccoli. Cook for 3 minutes, then pour in tamari sauce and mix well. Serve immediately.

N.V.: (per serving) Cal. 280 | Fat 12g | Carb. 10g | Prot. 32g

QUINOA & ROASTED RED PEPPER STUFFED PEPPERS

P.T.: 10 minutes (preparation), 20 minutes (cooking)

Ingr.:
- 1 large bell pepper, halved
- ½ cup cooked quinoa
- ¼ cup roasted red peppers, chopped
- 1 tbsp feta cheese
- ½ tsp dried oregano
- 1 tsp olive oil

Serv.: 2

Method of Cooking: Baking

Procedure:

Preheat oven to 375°F. Mix quinoa, roasted red peppers, feta cheese, oregano, and olive oil in a bowl. Stuff mixture into bell pepper halves and bake for 20 minutes until tender. Serve warm.

N.V.: (per serving) Cal. 220 | Fat 8g | Carb. 24g | Prot. 8g

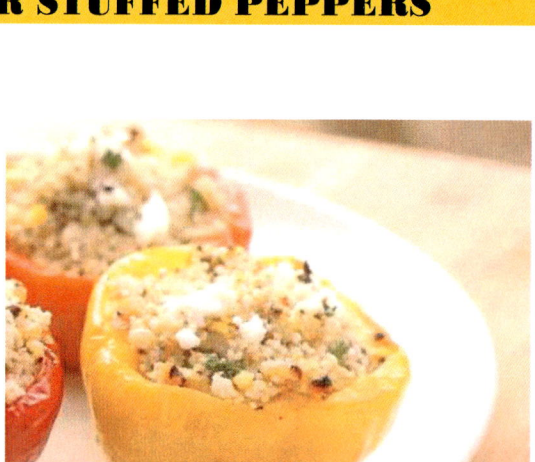

SPINACH & RICOTTA ZUCCHINI ROLL-UPS

P.T.: 10 minutes (preparation), 15 minutes (cooking)

Ingr.:
- 1 medium zucchini, sliced thin
- ½ cup ricotta cheese
- ½ cup fresh spinach, chopped
- ¼ tsp garlic powder
- 1 tbsp grated Parmesan
- 1 tsp olive oil

Serv.: 2

Method of Cooking: Baking

Procedure:

Preheat oven to 375°F. Mix ricotta cheese, spinach, garlic powder, and Parmesan in a bowl. Spread mixture onto zucchini slices, roll them up, and place in a baking dish. Drizzle with olive oil and bake for 15 minutes. Serve warm.

N.V.: (per serving) Cal. 180 | Fat 10g | Carb. 8g | Prot. 12g

ALMOND-CRUSTED TILAPIA WITH STEAMED GREEN BEANS

P.T.: 10 minutes (preparation), 10 minutes (cooking)

Ingr.:
- 2 small tilapia fillets
- 2 tbsp almond flour
- 1 tsp lemon zest
- ½ tsp garlic powder
- 1 tbsp olive oil
- 1 cup green beans

Serv.: 2

Method of Cooking: Pan-searing, steaming

Procedure:

Mix almond flour, lemon zest, and garlic powder. Coat tilapia fillets with the mixture. Heat olive oil in a skillet over medium heat and cook tilapia for 3-4 minutes per side until golden. Steam green beans for 5 minutes and serve alongside the fish.

N.V.: (per serving) Cal. 280 | Fat 12g | Carb. 10g | Prot. 32g

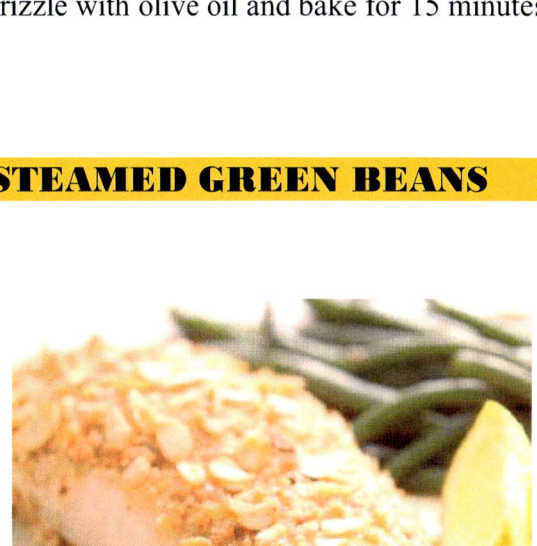

GREEK YOGURT & DILL EGG SALAD ON WHOLE WHEAT CRACKERS

P.T.: 5 minutes (preparation), 0 minutes (cooking)

Ingr.:
- 2 hard-boiled eggs, chopped
- ¼ cup plain Greek yogurt
- ½ tsp Dijon mustard
- 1 tsp chopped fresh dill
- ¼ tsp black pepper
- 4 whole wheat crackers

Serv.: 2

Method of Cooking: No-cook

Procedure:

Mix chopped eggs, Greek yogurt, Dijon mustard, dill, and black pepper in a bowl. Spoon mixture onto whole wheat crackers and serve immediately.

N.V.: (per serving) Cal. 220 | Fat 12g | Carb. 14g | Prot. 14g

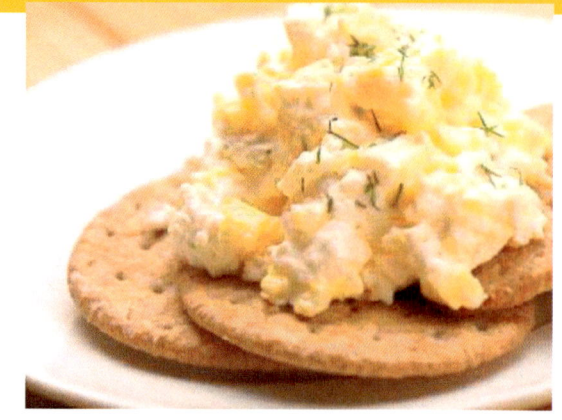

Chapter 4: Nourishing Dinners for Maximum Satisfaction

GARLIC BUTTER BAKED COD WITH ROASTED BRUSSELS SPROUTS

P .T.: 10 minutes (preparation), 15 minutes (cooking)

Ingr.:
- 2 small cod fillets
- 1 cup Brussels sprouts, halved
- 1 tbsp unsalted butter, melted
- 1 tsp minced garlic
- ½ tsp lemon zest
- ¼ tsp salt

Serv.: 2

Method of Cooking: Baking

Procedure:

Preheat oven to 375°F. Toss Brussels sprouts with half the melted butter, minced garlic, and salt, then spread onto a baking sheet. Roast for 10 minutes. Place cod fillets on the same sheet, brush with remaining butter and sprinkle with lemon zest. Bake for an additional 5 minutes or until cod flakes easily. Serve warm.

N.V.: (per serving) Cal. 250 | Fat 9g | Carb. 8g | Prot. 35g

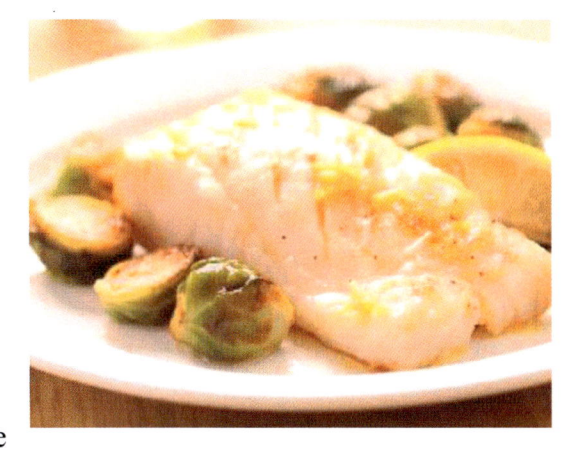

LEMON HERB GRILLED CHICKEN WITH CAULIFLOWER MASH

P.T.: 10 minutes (preparation), 15 minutes (cooking)

Ingr.:
- 2 small boneless chicken breasts
- 1 cup cauliflower florets
- 1 tbsp olive oil
- 1 tsp lemon juice
- ½ tsp dried thyme
- ¼ tsp salt

Serv.: 2

Method of Cooking: Grilling, steaming

Procedure:

Rub chicken breasts with olive oil, lemon juice, dried thyme, and salt. Grill over medium heat for 5 minutes per side until cooked through. Meanwhile, steam cauliflower florets until tender, then mash until smooth. Serve grilled chicken over mashed cauliflower.

N.V.: (per serving) Cal. 280 | Fat 10g | Carb. 6g | Prot. 38g

SPAGHETTI SQUASH WITH TURKEY BOLOGNESE

P.T.: 10 minutes (preparation), 25 minutes (cooking)

Ingr.:
- 1 small spaghetti squash, halved
- ½ cup ground turkey
- ½ cup crushed tomatoes
- ½ tsp dried oregano
- 1 tsp olive oil
- ¼ tsp black pepper

Serv.: 2

Method of Cooking: Roasting, stovetop

Procedure:

Preheat oven to 400°F. Place spaghetti squash halves cut side down on a baking sheet and roast for 20 minutes until fork-tender. Meanwhile, heat olive oil in a skillet over medium heat and cook ground turkey until browned. Add crushed tomatoes, oregano, and black pepper, then simmer for 5 minutes. Scrape spaghetti squash into strands and top with turkey bolognese.

N.V.: (per serving) Cal. 290 | Fat 12g | Carb. 20g | Prot. 28g

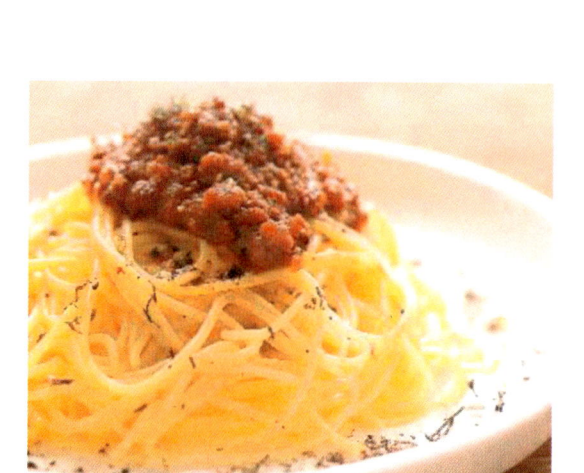

BALSAMIC GLAZED SALMON WITH SAUTÉED SPINACH

P.T.: 5 minutes (preparation), 15 minutes (cooking)

Ingr.:
- 2 small salmon fillets
- 1 tbsp balsamic vinegar
- 1 tsp olive oil
- 1 cup fresh spinach
- ¼ tsp garlic powder
- ¼ tsp salt

Serv.: 2

Method of Cooking: Baking, sautéing

Procedure:

Preheat oven to 375°F. Brush salmon fillets with balsamic vinegar and bake for 12 minutes. Meanwhile, heat olive oil in a skillet and sauté spinach with garlic powder and salt for 3 minutes until wilted. Serve salmon with sautéed spinach.

N.V.: (per serving) Cal. 320 | Fat 18g | Carb. 4g | Prot. 34g

STUFFED BELL PEPPERS WITH QUINOA & GROUND TURKEY

P.T.: 10 minutes (preparation), 20 minutes (cooking)

Ingr.:
- 1 large bell pepper, halved
- ½ cup cooked quinoa
- ½ cup ground turkey
- ½ tsp cumin
- 1 tsp olive oil
- ¼ tsp salt

Serv.: 2

Method of Cooking: Baking

Procedure:

Preheat oven to 375°F. Heat olive oil in a skillet and cook ground turkey with cumin and salt until browned. Mix with cooked quinoa, then stuff into bell pepper halves. Bake for 20 minutes until peppers are tender. Serve warm.

N.V.: (per serving) Cal. 260 | Fat 10g | Carb. 18g | Prot. 25g

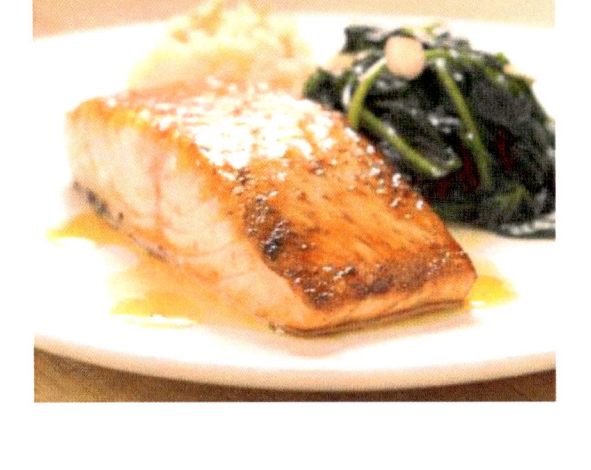

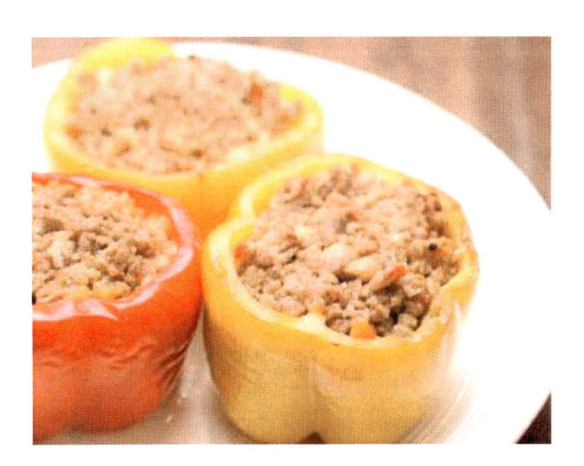

ZUCCHINI NOODLES WITH PESTO & GRILLED SHRIMP

P.T.: 10 minutes (preparation), 5 minutes (cooking)

Ingr.:
- 1 medium zucchini, spiralized
- 6 medium shrimp, peeled and deveined
- 1 tbsp basil pesto
- 1 tsp olive oil
- ¼ tsp black pepper
- ¼ tsp red pepper flakes

Serv.: 2

Method of Cooking: Grilling, sautéing

Procedure:

Heat olive oil in a grill pan and cook shrimp for 2 minutes per side until opaque. Sauté zucchini noodles for 2 minutes, then toss with basil pesto and black pepper. Serve topped with grilled shrimp and a sprinkle of red pepper flakes.

N.V.: (per serving) Cal. 240 | Fat 12g | Carb. 10g | Prot. 26g

SLOW COOKER CHICKEN & VEGETABLE STEW

P.T.: 10 minutes (preparation), 4 hours (cooking)

Ingr.:
- 2 small boneless chicken thighs
- ½ cup diced carrots
- ½ cup chopped celery
- 2 cups low-sodium chicken broth
- ½ tsp dried thyme
- ¼ tsp salt

Serv.: 2

Method of Cooking: Slow cooking

Procedure:

Place chicken, carrots, celery, broth, thyme, and salt in a slow cooker. Cover and cook on low for 4 hours until chicken is tender. Shred chicken with a fork before serving.

N.V.: (per serving) Cal. 270 | Fat 8g | Carb. 14g | Prot. 36g

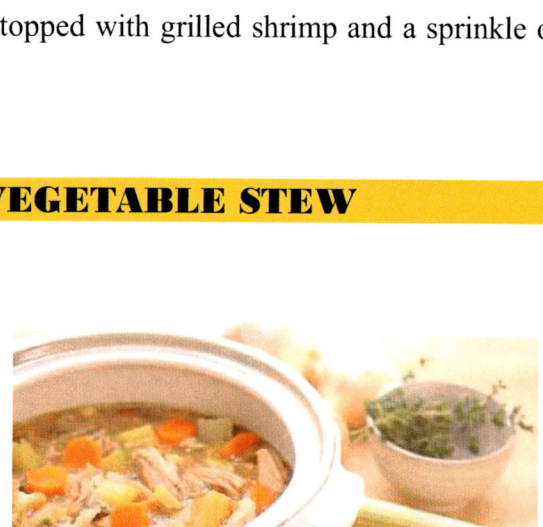

CAULIFLOWER CRUST PIZZA WITH TOMATO & MOZZARELLA

P.T.: 15 minutes (preparation), 20 minutes (cooking)

Ingr.:
- 1 cup riced cauliflower
- ½ cup shredded mozzarella cheese
- 1 egg
- ½ cup tomato sauce
- ½ tsp dried basil
- ¼ tsp garlic powder

Serv.: 2

Method of Cooking: Baking

Procedure:

Preheat oven to 400°F. Mix riced cauliflower, mozzarella, and egg into a dough. Press onto a baking sheet and bake for 10 minutes. Spread tomato sauce on top, sprinkle with basil and garlic powder, then bake for another 10 minutes. Serve warm.

N.V.: (per serving) Cal. 290 | Fat 14g | Carb. 18g | Prot. 22g

BEEF & MUSHROOM STIR-FRY WITH TAMARI SAUCE

P.T.: 10 minutes (preparation), 10 minutes (cooking)

Ingr.:
- 4 oz lean beef, sliced thin
- ½ cup sliced mushrooms
- 1 tbsp low-sodium tamari sauce
- 1 tsp sesame oil
- ¼ tsp black pepper
- ½ tsp grated ginger

Serv.: 2

Method of Cooking: Stir-frying

Procedure:

Heat sesame oil in a skillet over medium heat. Add beef and cook for 3 minutes until browned. Stir in mushrooms, ginger, black pepper, and tamari sauce. Cook for another 5 minutes until mushrooms are tender. Serve warm.

N.V.: (per serving) Cal. 280 | Fat 12g | Carb. 6g | Prot. 34g

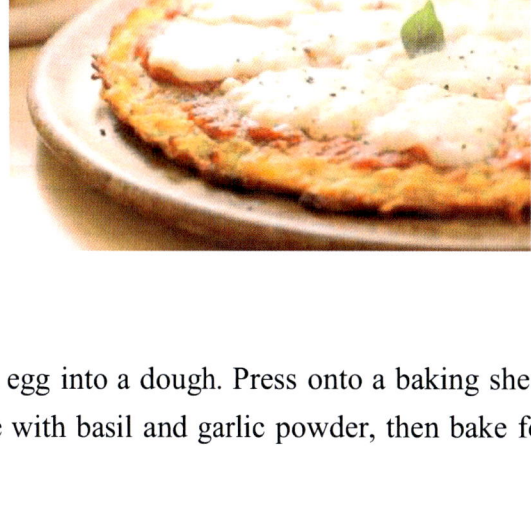

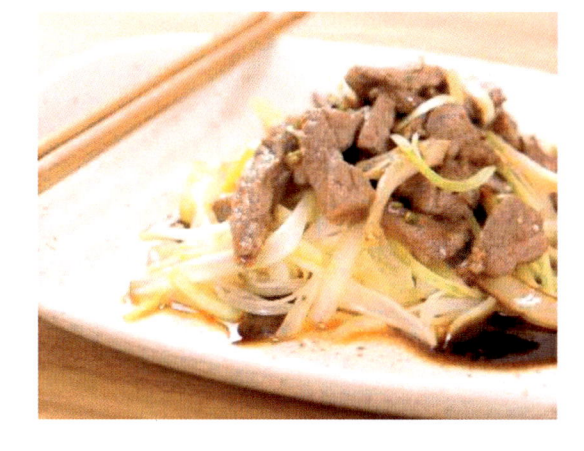

MEDITERRANEAN BAKED EGGPLANT WITH FETA & OLIVES

P.T.: 10 minutes (preparation), 20 minutes (cooking)

Ingr.:
- 1 small eggplant, sliced
- ¼ cup crumbled feta cheese
- 6 black olives, sliced
- 1 tbsp olive oil
- ½ tsp dried oregano
- ¼ tsp salt

Serv.: 2

Method of Cooking: Baking

Procedure:

Preheat oven to 375°F. Brush eggplant slices with olive oil and sprinkle with oregano and salt. Bake for 15 minutes, then top with feta and olives. Bake for another 5 minutes. Serve warm.

N.V.: (per serving) Cal. 240 | Fat 14g | Carb. 12g | Prot. 10g

HERB-ROASTED CHICKEN THIGHS WITH GARLIC GREEN BEANS

P.T.: 10 minutes (preparation), 25 minutes (cooking)

Ingr.:
- 2 small bone-in, skin-on chicken thighs
- 1 cup green beans, trimmed
- 1 tbsp olive oil
- ½ tsp dried rosemary
- ½ tsp garlic powder
- ¼ tsp salt

Serv.: 2

Method of Cooking: Roasting

Procedure:

Preheat oven to 400°F. Rub chicken thighs with half the olive oil, rosemary, garlic powder, and salt. Place on a baking sheet and roast for 20 minutes. Toss green beans with remaining olive oil and add to the sheet. Roast for an additional 5 minutes until chicken is crispy and green beans are tender. Serve warm.

N.V.: (per serving) Cal. 320 | Fat 18g | Carb. 6g | Prot. 34g

LENTIL & SWEET POTATO CURRY WITH COCONUT MILK

P.T.: 10 minutes (preparation), 20 minutes (cooking)

Ingr.:
- ½ cup dry lentils

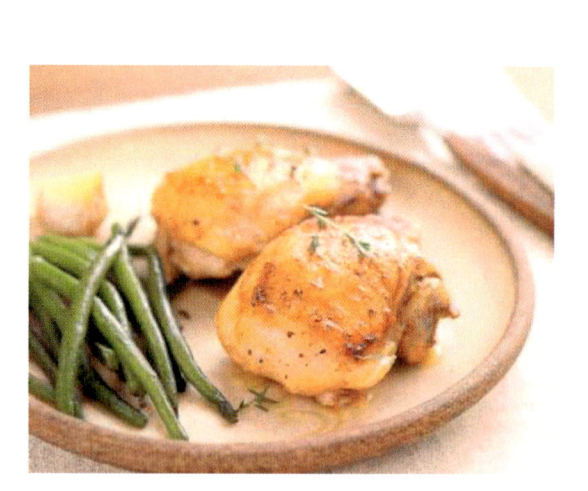

- ½ cup diced sweet potatoes
- ½ cup coconut milk
- 1 tsp curry powder
- 1 cup low-sodium vegetable broth
- ¼ tsp black pepper

Serv.: 2

Method of Cooking: Stovetop

Procedure:

In a saucepan over medium heat, combine lentils, sweet potatoes, vegetable broth, curry powder, and black pepper. Simmer for 15 minutes until lentils are tender. Stir in coconut milk and cook for another 5 minutes. Serve warm.

N.V.: (per serving) Cal. 280 | Fat 10g | Carb. 34g | Prot. 14g

PARMESAN-CRUSTED TILAPIA WITH ROASTED BROCCOLI

P.T.: 10 minutes (preparation), 15 minutes (cooking)

Ingr.:
- 2 small tilapia fillets
- 2 tbsp grated Parmesan cheese
- 1 tsp olive oil
- ½ cup broccoli florets
- ½ tsp garlic powder
- ¼ tsp salt

Serv.: 2

Method of Cooking: Baking

Procedure:

Preheat oven to 375°F. Brush tilapia fillets with olive oil, then coat with Parmesan and garlic powder. Place on a baking sheet and roast for 15 minutes. Toss broccoli with salt and roast on the same sheet for the last 10 minutes. Serve warm.

N.V.: (per serving) Cal. 270 | Fat 12g | Carb. 6g | Prot. 34g

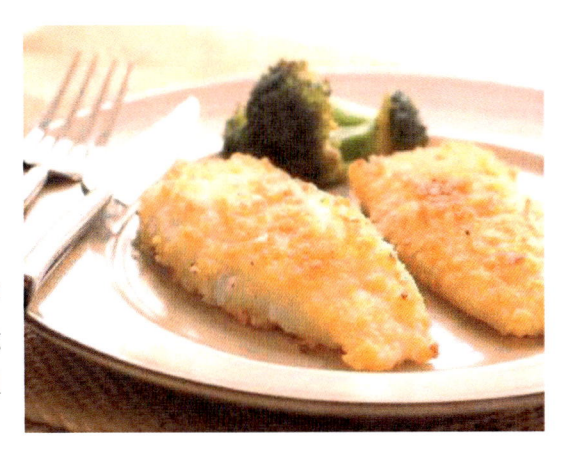

SPINACH & RICOTTA STUFFED CHICKEN BREAST

P.T.: 10 minutes (preparation), 25 minutes (cooking)

Ingr.:
- 2 small boneless, skinless chicken breasts
- ½ cup fresh spinach, chopped
- ¼ cup ricotta cheese
- 1 tsp olive oil
- ½ tsp garlic powder
- ¼ tsp black pepper

Serv.: 2

Method of Cooking: Baking

Procedure:

Preheat oven to 375°F. Slice a pocket into each chicken breast. Mix ricotta, spinach, garlic powder, and black pepper in a bowl. Stuff mixture into the chicken pockets. Brush with olive oil and bake for 25 minutes until cooked through. Serve warm.

N.V.: (per serving) Cal. 310 | Fat 12g | Carb. 4g | Prot. 42g

GRILLED PORTOBELLO MUSHROOMS WITH GARLIC & PARMESAN

P.T.: 10 minutes (preparation), 10 minutes (cooking)

Ingr.:
- 2 large Portobello mushrooms
- 1 tbsp olive oil
- ½ tsp minced garlic
- 2 tbsp grated Parmesan cheese
- ½ tsp balsamic vinegar
- ¼ tsp black pepper

Serv.: 2

Method of Cooking: Grilling

Procedure:

Brush mushrooms with olive oil, garlic, balsamic vinegar, and black pepper. Grill over medium heat for 5 minutes per side until tender. Sprinkle with Parmesan cheese before serving.

N.V.: (per serving) Cal. 180 | Fat 12g | Carb. 6g | Prot. 10g

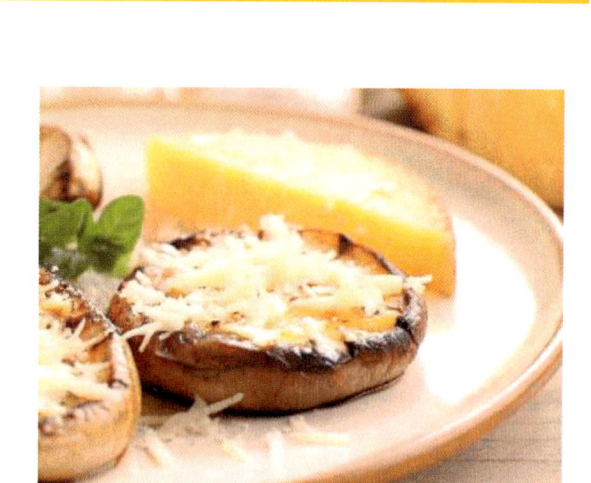

CAULIFLOWER FRIED RICE WITH SHRIMP & SCRAMBLED EGG

P.T.: 10 minutes (preparation), 10 minutes (cooking)

Ingr.:
- ½ cup riced cauliflower
- 6 medium shrimp, peeled and deveined
- 1 large egg, beaten
- 1 tbsp low-sodium soy sauce
- 1 tsp sesame oil
- ¼ tsp black pepper

Serv.: 2

Method of Cooking: Stir-frying

Procedure:

Heat sesame oil in a skillet over medium heat. Cook shrimp until pink, about 3 minutes. Push shrimp to the side and scramble the egg in the same pan. Stir in riced cauliflower, soy sauce, and black pepper. Cook for another 5 minutes, stirring frequently. Serve warm.

N.V.: (per serving) Cal. 220 | Fat 9g | Carb. 8g | Prot. 26g

TURKEY & ZUCCHINI MEATLOAF WITH MASHED CAULIFLOWER

P.T.: 10 minutes (preparation), 30 minutes (cooking)

Ingr.:
- ½ lb ground turkey
- ½ cup grated zucchini
- 1 large egg
- ½ tsp dried oregano
- 1 tsp olive oil
- 1 cup steamed cauliflower

Serv.: 2

Method of Cooking: Baking, steaming

Procedure:

Preheat oven to 375°F. Mix ground turkey, zucchini, egg, oregano, and half the olive oil. Form into two small loaves and bake for 30 minutes. Meanwhile, mash steamed cauliflower with remaining olive oil. Serve meatloaf with mashed cauliflower.

N.V.: (per serving) Cal. 320 | Fat 12g | Carb. 10g | Prot. 38g

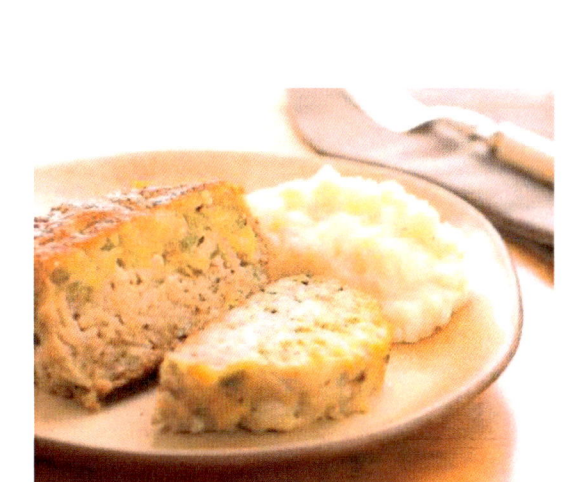

CABBAGE STIR-FRY WITH GROUND TURKEY & GINGER

P.T.: 10 minutes (preparation), 10 minutes (cooking)

Ingr.:
- ½ cup shredded cabbage
- ½ cup ground turkey
- 1 tsp grated ginger
- 1 tbsp low-sodium soy sauce
- 1 tsp sesame oil
- ¼ tsp red pepper flakes

Serv.: 2

Method of Cooking: Stir-frying

Procedure:

Heat sesame oil in a skillet over medium heat. Brown ground turkey, then stir in shredded cabbage, ginger, soy sauce, and red pepper flakes. Cook for another 5 minutes, stirring occasionally. Serve warm.

N.V.: (per serving) Cal. 250 | Fat 10g | Carb. 8g | Prot. 30g

CREAMY AVOCADO & CHICKEN ZOODLE BOWL

P.T.: 10 minutes (preparation), 5 minutes (cooking)

Ingr.:
- 1 medium zucchini, spiralized
- ½ cup cooked shredded chicken
- ½ small avocado, mashed
- 1 tsp lemon juice
- ¼ tsp black pepper
- 1 tsp olive oil

Serv.: 2

Method of Cooking: Sautéing

Procedure:

Heat olive oil in a skillet over medium heat. Sauté zucchini noodles for 2 minutes. Toss with shredded chicken, mashed avocado, lemon juice, and black pepper. Serve immediately.

N.V.: (per serving) Cal. 260 | Fat 14g | Carb. 8g | Prot. 28g

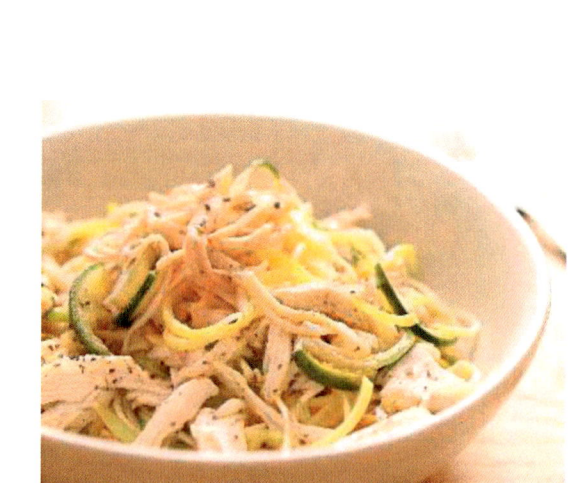

ROASTED BUTTERNUT SQUASH & KALE BOWL WITH QUINOA

P.T.: 10 minutes (preparation), 20 minutes (cooking)

Ingr.:
- ½ cup cubed butternut squash
- 1 cup chopped kale
- ½ cup cooked quinoa
- 1 tbsp olive oil
- ½ tsp cinnamon
- ¼ tsp salt

Serv.: 2

Method of Cooking: Roasting, stovetop

Procedure:

Preheat oven to 400°F. Toss butternut squash with olive oil and cinnamon, then roast for 20 minutes. Meanwhile, sauté kale in a pan with a little water until wilted. Mix with cooked quinoa and roasted squash. Serve warm.

N.V.: (per serving) Cal. 280 | Fat 10g | Carb. 34g | Prot. 8g

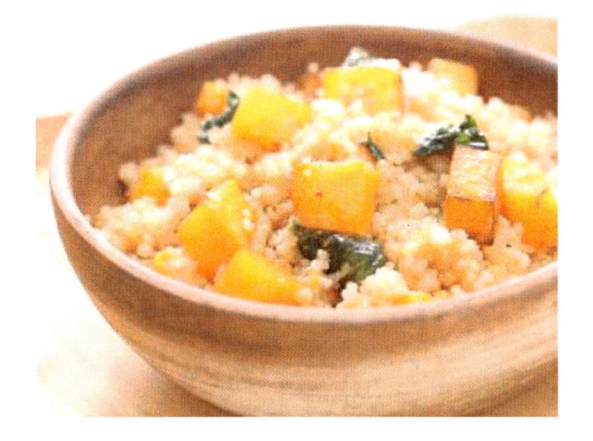

Chapter 5: Delicious Sides and Vegetables That Support Healthy Blood Sugar

GARLIC ROASTED BRUSSELS SPROUTS WITH ALMONDS

P.T.: 5 minutes (preparation), 20 minutes (cooking)

Ingr.:
- 1 cup Brussels sprouts, halved
- 1 tbsp olive oil
- 1 tsp minced garlic
- 2 tbsp sliced almonds
- ¼ tsp black pepper
- ¼ tsp salt

Serv.: 2

Method of Cooking: Roasting

Procedure:

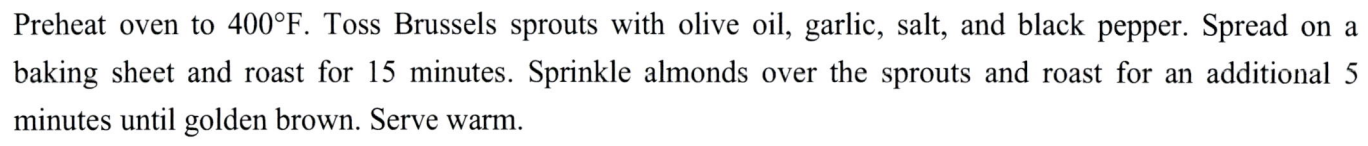

Preheat oven to 400°F. Toss Brussels sprouts with olive oil, garlic, salt, and black pepper. Spread on a baking sheet and roast for 15 minutes. Sprinkle almonds over the sprouts and roast for an additional 5 minutes until golden brown. Serve warm.

N.V.: (per serving) Cal. 180 | Fat 12g | Carb. 10g | Prot. 6g

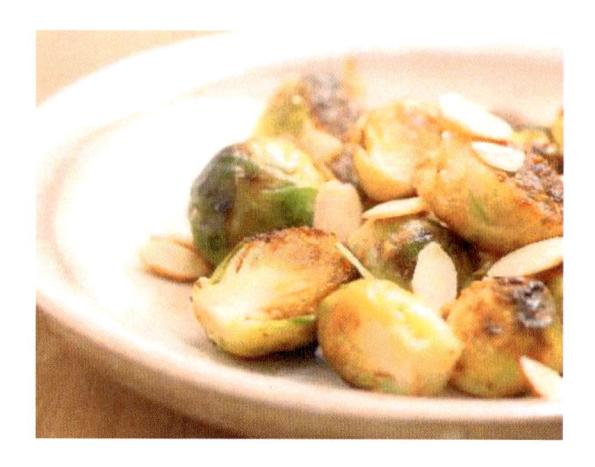

SAUTÉED ZUCCHINI & MUSHROOMS WITH PARMESAN

P.T.: 5 minutes (preparation), 10 minutes (cooking)

Ingr.:
- 1 medium zucchini, sliced
- ½ cup sliced mushrooms
- 1 tbsp olive oil
- 1 tbsp grated Parmesan cheese
- ¼ tsp garlic powder
- ¼ tsp black pepper

Serv.: 2

Method of Cooking: Sautéing

Procedure:

Heat olive oil in a skillet over medium heat. Add zucchini and mushrooms, sautéing for 8 minutes until tender. Sprinkle with garlic powder, black pepper, and Parmesan cheese. Stir gently and serve warm.

N.V.: (per serving) Cal. 140 | Fat 10g | Carb. 7g | Prot. 5g

BALSAMIC GLAZED ROASTED CARROTS & ONIONS

P.T.: 5 minutes (preparation), 25 minutes (cooking)

Ingr.:
- 1 cup baby carrots
- ½ small red onion, sliced
- 1 tbsp balsamic vinegar
- 1 tbsp olive oil
- ¼ tsp salt
- ¼ tsp dried thyme

Serv.: 2

Method of Cooking: Roasting

Procedure:

Preheat oven to 400°F. Toss carrots and onions with balsamic vinegar, olive oil, salt, and thyme. Spread on a baking sheet and roast for 25 minutes until caramelized and tender. Serve warm.

N.V.: (per serving) Cal. 160 | Fat 8g | Carb. 18g | Prot. 2g

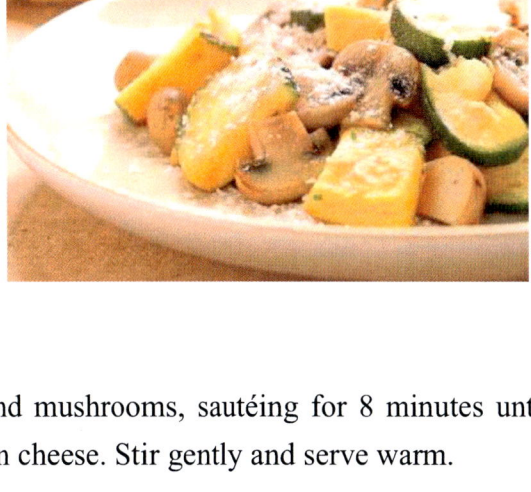

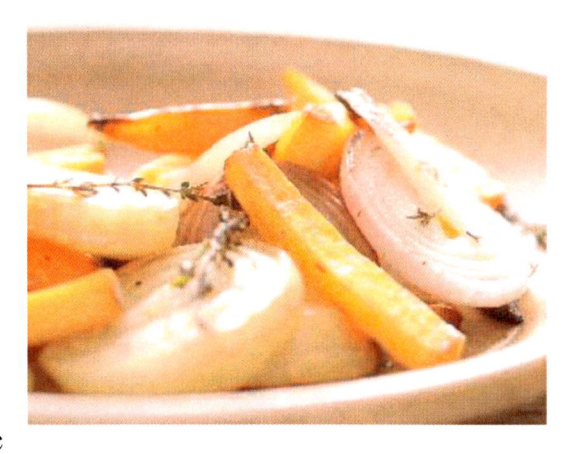

SPICY CAULIFLOWER RICE WITH CILANTRO & LIME

P.T.: 5 minutes (preparation), 10 minutes (cooking)

Ingr.:
- 1 cup riced cauliflower
- ½ tsp ground cumin
- ½ tsp red pepper flakes
- 1 tbsp chopped cilantro
- 1 tsp olive oil
- Juice of ½ lime

Serv.: 2

Method of Cooking: Sautéing

Procedure:

Heat olive oil in a skillet over medium heat. Add riced cauliflower, cumin, and red pepper flakes, sautéing for 5 minutes. Remove from heat and stir in lime juice and cilantro. Serve warm.

N.V.: (per serving) Cal. 110 | Fat 6g | Carb. 10g | Prot. 3g

CREAMY AVOCADO & CUCUMBER SALAD WITH LEMON DRESSING

P.T.: 5 minutes (preparation), 0 minutes (cooking)

Ingr.:
- ½ avocado, diced
- ½ small cucumber, sliced
- 1 tsp lemon juice
- 1 tsp olive oil
- ¼ tsp black pepper
- ¼ tsp dried dill

Serv.: 2

Method of Cooking: No-cook

Procedure:

In a bowl, combine avocado, cucumber, lemon juice, olive oil, black pepper, and dill. Toss gently and serve chilled.

N.V.: (per serving) Cal. 160 | Fat 12g | Carb. 8g | Prot. 2g

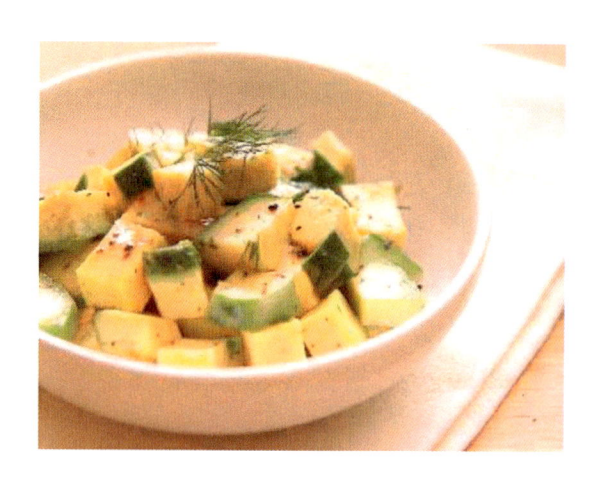

ROASTED SWEET POTATO WEDGES WITH PAPRIKA

P.T.: 5 minutes (preparation), 25 minutes (cooking)

Ingr.:
- 1 small sweet potato, cut into wedges
- 1 tbsp olive oil
- ½ tsp smoked paprika
- ¼ tsp salt
- ¼ tsp black pepper
- ¼ tsp garlic powder

Serv.: 2

Method of Cooking: Roasting

Procedure:

Preheat oven to 400°F. Toss sweet potato wedges with olive oil, paprika, salt, black pepper, and garlic powder. Spread on a baking sheet and roast for 25 minutes, flipping halfway through. Serve warm.

N.V.: (per serving) Cal. 190 | Fat 8g | Carb. 26g | Prot. 3g

SAUTÉED KALE WITH GARLIC & OLIVE OIL

P.T.: 5 minutes (preparation), 5 minutes (cooking)

Ingr.:
- 1 cup kale, chopped
- 1 tsp olive oil
- ½ tsp minced garlic
- ¼ tsp red pepper flakes
- ¼ tsp salt
- 1 tsp lemon juice

Serv.: 2

Method of Cooking: Sautéing

Procedure:

Heat olive oil in a skillet over medium heat. Add garlic and red pepper flakes, sautéing for 1 minute. Stir in kale and salt, cooking for 4 minutes until wilted. Remove from heat and drizzle with lemon juice. Serve warm.

N.V.: (per serving) Cal. 100 | Fat 6g | Carb. 7g | Prot. 3g

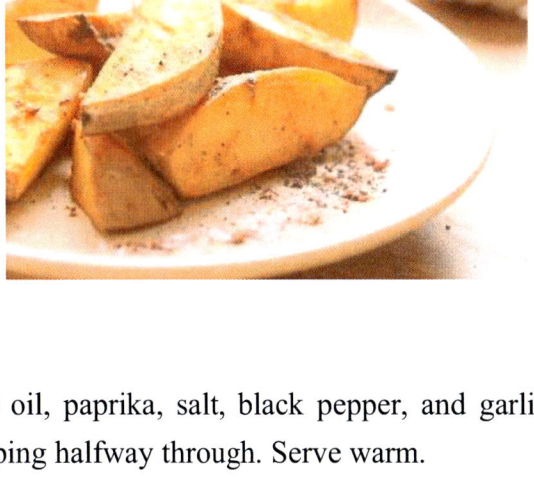

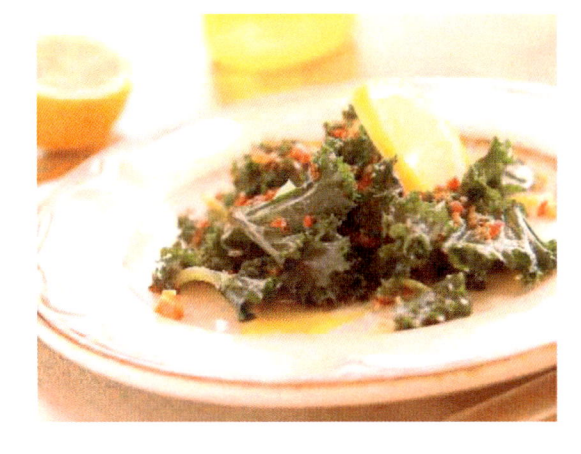

GRILLED ASPARAGUS WITH LEMON & FETA

P.T.: 5 minutes (preparation), 8 minutes (cooking)

Ingr.:
- 6 asparagus spears
- 1 tbsp olive oil
- 1 tsp lemon juice
- 1 tbsp crumbled feta cheese
- ¼ tsp salt
- ¼ tsp black pepper

Serv.: 2

Method of Cooking: Grilling

Procedure:

Brush asparagus spears with olive oil, salt, and black pepper. Grill over medium heat for 6-8 minutes, turning occasionally. Transfer to a plate and drizzle with lemon juice. Sprinkle with feta before serving.

N.V.: (per serving) Cal. 120 | Fat 8g | Carb. 5g | Prot. 3g

HERB-ROASTED BUTTERNUT SQUASH WITH WALNUTS

P.T.: 5 minutes (preparation), 25 minutes (cooking)

Ingr.:
- ½ cup cubed butternut squash
- 1 tbsp olive oil
- ¼ tsp ground cinnamon
- ¼ tsp dried rosemary
- 1 tbsp chopped walnuts
- ¼ tsp salt

Serv.: 2

Method of Cooking: Roasting

Procedure:

Preheat oven to 400°F. Toss butternut squash with olive oil, cinnamon, rosemary, and salt. Spread on a baking sheet and roast for 20 minutes. Sprinkle with walnuts and roast for an additional 5 minutes. Serve warm.

N.V.: (per serving) Cal. 180 | Fat 10g | Carb. 18g | Prot. 3g

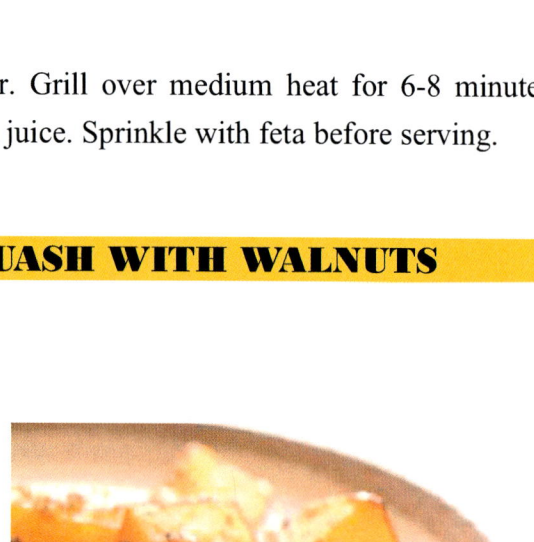

STEAMED GREEN BEANS WITH TOASTED SESAME SEEDS

P.T.: 5 minutes (preparation), 5 minutes (cooking)

Ingr.:
- 1 cup green beans, trimmed
- 1 tsp olive oil
- 1 tsp toasted sesame seeds
- ¼ tsp black pepper
- ¼ tsp salt
- ½ tsp lemon zest

Serv.: 2

Method of Cooking: Steaming

Procedure:

Steam green beans for 5 minutes until tender. Transfer to a bowl and toss with olive oil, sesame seeds, black pepper, salt, and lemon zest. Serve warm.

N.V.: (per serving) Cal. 100 | Fat 6g | Carb. 8g | Prot. 2g

MASHED CAULIFLOWER WITH GARLIC & CHIVES

P.T.: 5 minutes (preparation), 10 minutes (cooking)

Ingr.:
- 1 cup cauliflower florets
- 1 tsp olive oil
- ½ tsp minced garlic
- 1 tbsp chopped chives
- ¼ tsp salt
- ¼ tsp black pepper

Serv.: 2

Method of Cooking: Steaming, blending

Procedure:

Steam cauliflower florets for 10 minutes until fork-tender. Transfer to a bowl and mash with olive oil, garlic, salt, and black pepper until smooth. Stir in chopped chives and serve warm.

N.V.: (per serving) Cal. 110 | Fat 6g | Carb. 9g | Prot. 3g

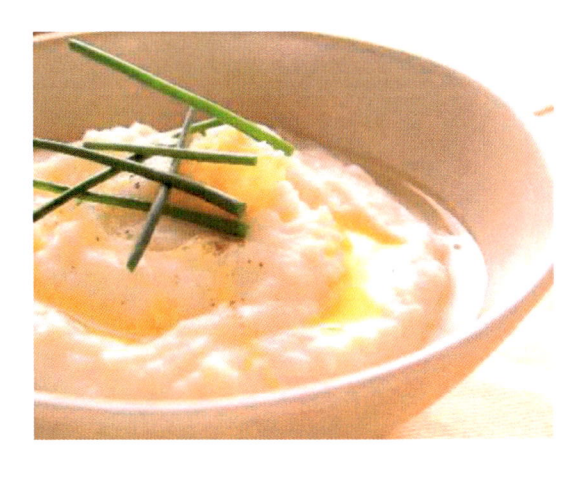

SPAGHETTI SQUASH WITH BASIL & CHERRY TOMATOES

P.T.: 5 minutes (preparation), 25 minutes (cooking)

Ingr.:
- 1 small spaghetti squash, halved
- ½ cup cherry tomatoes, halved
- 1 tbsp olive oil
- 1 tsp dried basil
- ¼ tsp garlic powder
- ¼ tsp salt

Serv.: 2

Method of Cooking: Roasting

Procedure:

Preheat oven to 400°F. Place spaghetti squash halves cut side down on a baking sheet and roast for 20 minutes until tender. Use a fork to scrape the strands into a bowl. Toss with olive oil, cherry tomatoes, dried basil, garlic powder, and salt. Serve warm.

N.V.: (per serving) Cal. 140 | Fat 7g | Carb. 15g | Prot. 3g

CRISPY BAKED EGGPLANT SLICES WITH ITALIAN HERBS

P.T.: 10 minutes (preparation), 20 minutes (cooking)

Ingr.:
- 1 small eggplant, sliced into rounds
- 1 tbsp olive oil
- 1 tbsp grated Parmesan cheese
- ½ tsp dried oregano
- ¼ tsp black pepper
- ¼ tsp salt

Serv.: 2

Method of Cooking: Baking

Procedure:

Preheat oven to 375°F. Brush eggplant slices with olive oil and sprinkle with Parmesan, oregano, black pepper, and salt. Arrange on a baking sheet and bake for 20 minutes until golden and crispy. Serve warm.

N.V.: (per serving) Cal. 150 | Fat 8g | Carb. 10g | Prot. 5g

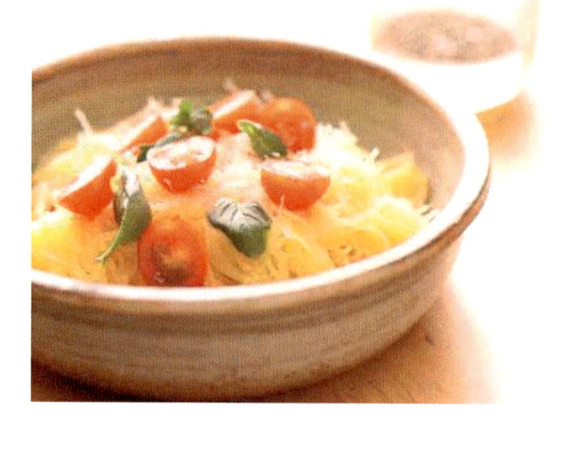

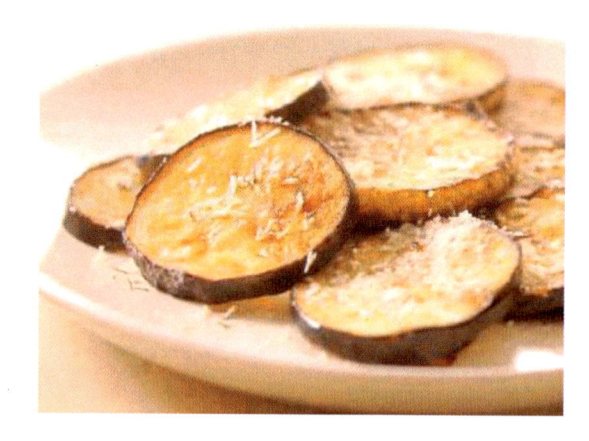

BROCCOLI & CHEDDAR STUFFED MUSHROOMS

P.T.: 5 minutes (preparation), 15 minutes (cooking)

Ingr.:
- 4 large white mushrooms, stems removed
- ½ cup chopped broccoli
- ¼ cup shredded cheddar cheese
- 1 tsp olive oil
- ¼ tsp garlic powder
- ¼ tsp salt

Serv.: 2

Method of Cooking: Baking

Procedure:

Preheat oven to 375°F. Sauté chopped broccoli with olive oil and garlic powder for 3 minutes. Mix with shredded cheddar cheese and salt. Stuff the mixture into mushroom caps and bake for 12 minutes until the cheese is melted and mushrooms are tender. Serve warm.

N.V.: (per serving) Cal. 180 | Fat 10g | Carb. 8g | Prot. 9g

MEDITERRANEAN CUCUMBER & CHICKPEA SALAD

P.T.: 5 minutes (preparation), 0 minutes (cooking)

Ingr.:
- ½ cup canned chickpeas, rinsed
- ½ small cucumber, diced
- 1 tbsp olive oil
- 1 tsp lemon juice
- ¼ tsp dried oregano
- ¼ tsp black pepper

Serv.: 2

Method of Cooking: No-cook

Procedure:

In a bowl, combine chickpeas, cucumber, olive oil, lemon juice, oregano, and black pepper. Toss gently and serve chilled.

N.V.: (per serving) Cal. 160 | Fat 8g | Carb. 14g | Prot. 6g

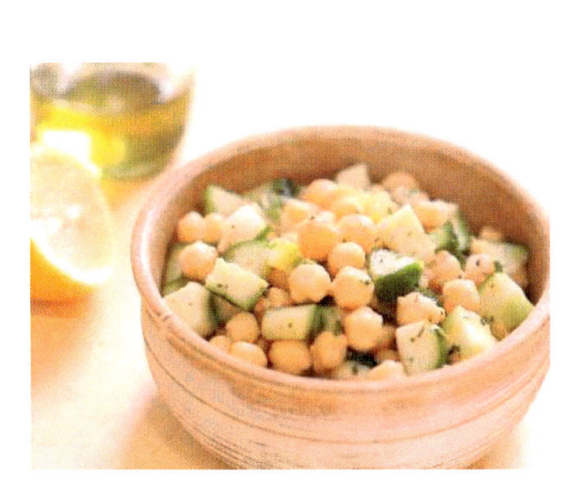

Chapter 6: Guilt-Free Desserts to Satisfy Your Sweet Tooth

DARK CHOCOLATE & ALMOND BUTTER CHIA PUDDING

P.T.: 5 minutes (preparation), 0 minutes (cooking)

Ingr.:
- 1 cup unsweetened almond milk
- 2 tbsp chia seeds
- 1 tbsp almond butter
- 1 tbsp unsweetened cocoa powder
- 1 tsp monk fruit sweetener
- ½ tsp vanilla extract

Serv.: 2

Method of Cooking: No-cook, refrigeration

Procedure:

In a bowl, whisk together almond milk, cocoa powder, almond butter, vanilla extract, and monk fruit sweetener until smooth. Stir in chia seeds and mix well. Let sit for 5 minutes, then stir again to prevent clumping. Cover and refrigerate for at least 3 hours or overnight. Stir before serving.

N.V.: (per serving) Cal. 190 | Fat 12g | Carb. 10g | Prot. 6g

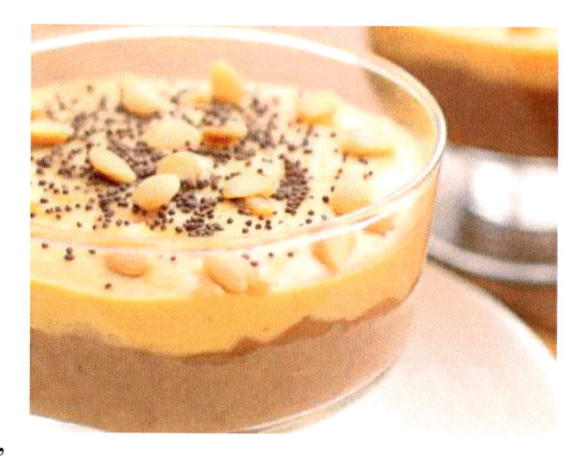

BAKED CINNAMON APPLES WITH WALNUTS & GREEK YOGURT

P.T.: 5 minutes (preparation), 20 minutes (cooking)

Ingr.:
- 1 small apple, sliced
- ½ tsp ground cinnamon
- 1 tsp unsalted butter, melted
- 1 tbsp chopped walnuts
- ¼ cup plain Greek yogurt
- 1 tsp monk fruit sweetener

Serv.: 2

Method of Cooking: Baking

Procedure:

Preheat oven to 375°F. Toss apple slices with melted butter, cinnamon, and monk fruit sweetener. Spread on a baking sheet and bake for 20 minutes until tender. Serve warm with a dollop of Greek yogurt and a sprinkle of walnuts.

N.V.: (per serving) Cal. 160 | Fat 6g | Carb. 20g | Prot. 5g

COCONUT FLOUR BLUEBERRY MUFFINS

P.T.: 5 minutes (preparation), 15 minutes (cooking)

Ingr.:
- ¼ cup coconut flour
- 1 large egg
- ¼ cup unsweetened almond milk
- ¼ cup fresh blueberries
- ½ tsp baking powder
- 1 tsp monk fruit sweetener

Serv.: 2

Method of Cooking: Baking

Procedure:

Preheat oven to 350°F. In a bowl, mix coconut flour, baking powder, and monk fruit sweetener. Whisk in egg and almond milk until smooth. Fold in blueberries. Pour batter into muffin cups and bake for 15 minutes. Let cool before serving.

N.V.: (per serving) Cal. 150 | Fat 8g | Carb. 10g | Prot. 5g

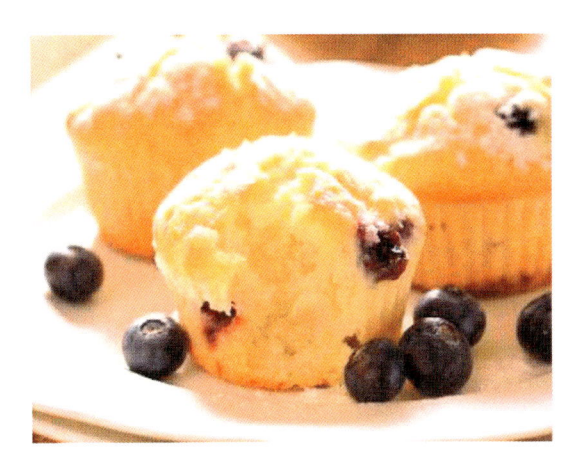

SUGAR-FREE CHOCOLATE AVOCADO MOUSSE

P.T.: 5 minutes (preparation), 0 minutes (cooking)

Ingr.:
- ½ ripe avocado
- 2 tbsp unsweetened cocoa powder
- 2 tbsp unsweetened almond milk
- 1 tsp monk fruit sweetener
- ½ tsp vanilla extract
- ¼ tsp cinnamon

Serv.: 2

Method of Cooking: Blending

Procedure:

In a blender, combine avocado, cocoa powder, almond milk, monk fruit sweetener, vanilla extract, and cinnamon. Blend until smooth and creamy. Chill for 10 minutes before serving.

N.V.: (per serving) Cal. 180 | Fat 12g | Carb. 8g | Prot. 3g

ALMOND FLOUR PEANUT BUTTER COOKIES

P.T.: 5 minutes (preparation), 12 minutes (cooking)

Ingr.:
- ½ cup almond flour
- 2 tbsp natural peanut butter
- 1 tbsp monk fruit sweetener
- ½ tsp baking powder
- ½ tsp vanilla extract
- 1 egg

Serv.: 2

Method of Cooking: Baking

Procedure:

Preheat oven to 350°F. In a bowl, mix almond flour, baking powder, and monk fruit sweetener. Stir in peanut butter, vanilla extract, and egg until a dough forms. Shape into small cookies and place on a baking sheet. Bake for 12 minutes until golden brown. Let cool before serving.

N.V.: (per serving) Cal. 190 | Fat 14g | Carb. 6g | Prot. 6g

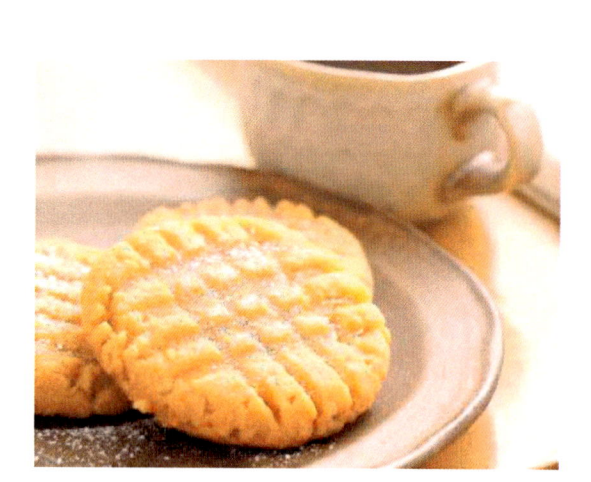

NO-BAKE COCONUT & CHIA ENERGY BITES

P.T.: 5 minutes (preparation), 0 minutes (cooking)

Ingr.:
- ¼ cup unsweetened shredded coconut
- 1 tbsp chia seeds
- 1 tbsp almond butter
- 1 tsp monk fruit sweetener
- ½ tsp vanilla extract
- 1 tsp water

Serv.: 2

Method of Cooking: No-cook, refrigeration

Procedure:

In a bowl, mix shredded coconut, chia seeds, almond butter, monk fruit sweetener, vanilla extract, and water until well combined. Roll into small balls and refrigerate for at least 20 minutes before serving.

N.V.: (per serving) Cal. 160 | Fat 12g | Carb. 7g | Prot. 3g

LEMON RICOTTA CHEESECAKE BARS

P.T.: 5 minutes (preparation), 20 minutes (cooking)

Ingr.:
- ½ cup ricotta cheese
- 1 large egg
- 1 tbsp almond flour
- 1 tbsp lemon juice
- 1 tsp monk fruit sweetener
- ½ tsp vanilla extract

Serv.: 2

Method of Cooking: Baking

Procedure:

Preheat oven to 350°F. In a bowl, whisk ricotta cheese, egg, almond flour, lemon juice, monk fruit sweetener, and vanilla extract until smooth. Pour into a greased baking dish and bake for 20 minutes. Let cool before slicing into bars.

N.V.: (per serving) Cal. 200 | Fat 12g | Carb. 8g | Prot. 10g

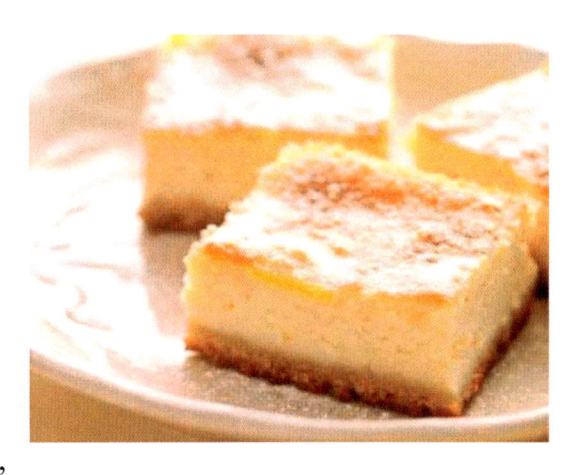

RASPBERRY & DARK CHOCOLATE FROZEN YOGURT BARK

P.T.: 5 minutes (preparation), 2 hours (freezing)

Ingr.:
- ½ cup plain Greek yogurt
- 1 tbsp unsweetened dark chocolate chips
- ¼ cup fresh raspberries
- 1 tsp monk fruit sweetener
- ½ tsp vanilla extract
- 1 tsp shredded coconut

Serv.: 2

Method of Cooking: Freezing

Procedure:

Mix Greek yogurt, vanilla extract, and monk fruit sweetener in a bowl. Spread evenly on a parchment-lined baking sheet. Sprinkle with raspberries, dark chocolate chips, and shredded coconut. Freeze for at least 2 hours. Break into pieces before serving.

N.V.: (per serving) Cal. 140 | Fat 6g | Carb. 12g | Prot. 8g

VANILLA CHIA & FLAXSEED PUDDING WITH BERRIES

P.T.: 5 minutes (preparation), 0 minutes (cooking)

Ingr.:
- 1 cup unsweetened almond milk
- 1 tbsp chia seeds
- 1 tbsp ground flaxseeds
- ½ tsp vanilla extract
- 1 tsp monk fruit sweetener
- ¼ cup fresh mixed berries

Serv.: 2

Method of Cooking: No-cook, refrigeration

Procedure:

In a bowl, whisk together almond milk, vanilla extract, monk fruit sweetener, chia seeds, and ground flaxseeds. Stir well and refrigerate for at least 3 hours or overnight. Before serving, top with fresh berries.

N.V.: (per serving) Cal. 150 | Fat 9g | Carb. 10g | Prot. 5g

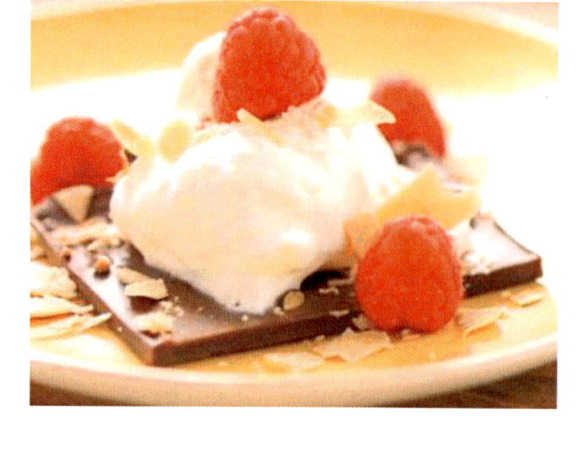

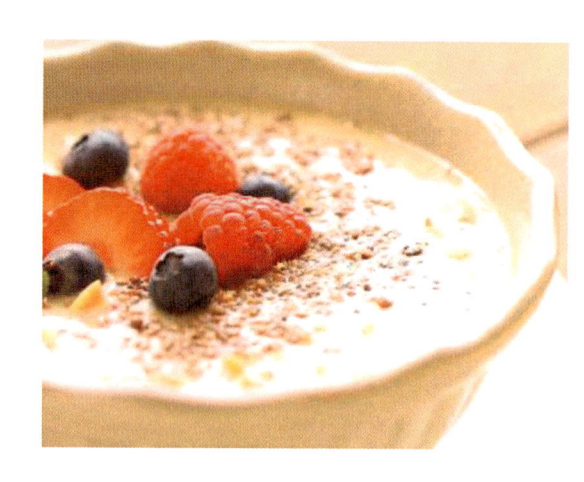

SPICED PUMPKIN & PECAN MUG CAKE

P.T.: 5 minutes (preparation), 2 minutes (cooking)

Ingr.:
- 2 tbsp almond flour
- 1 tbsp pumpkin purée
- 1 tbsp chopped pecans
- ½ tsp pumpkin spice
- 1 tsp monk fruit sweetener
- 1 large egg

Serv.: 2

Method of Cooking: Microwave

Procedure:

In a microwave-safe mug, mix almond flour, pumpkin purée, pumpkin spice, monk fruit sweetener, and egg until smooth. Stir in chopped pecans. Microwave for 2 minutes until set. Let cool slightly before serving.

N.V.: (per serving) Cal. 180 | Fat 12g | Carb. 8g | Prot. 7g

CHOCOLATE ZUCCHINI BROWNIES (LOW-CARB)

P.T.: 5 minutes (preparation), 20 minutes (cooking)

Ingr.:
- ½ cup grated zucchini
- ¼ cup almond flour
- 2 tbsp unsweetened cocoa powder
- 1 large egg
- 1 tbsp monk fruit sweetener
- ½ tsp baking powder

Serv.: 2

Method of Cooking: Baking

Procedure:

Preheat oven to 350°F. In a bowl, mix grated zucchini, almond flour, cocoa powder, baking powder, and monk fruit sweetener. Stir in the egg until a batter forms. Pour into a small greased baking dish and bake for 20 minutes until set. Let cool before serving.

N.V.: (per serving) Cal. 160 | Fat 10g | Carb. 9g | Prot. 6g

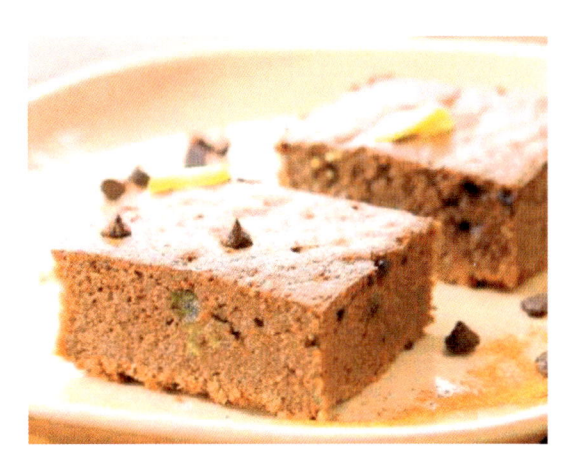

SUGAR-FREE BANANA & WALNUT ICE CREAM

P.T.: 5 minutes (preparation), 2 hours (freezing)

Ingr.:
- 1 ripe banana, sliced and frozen
- ¼ cup unsweetened almond milk
- 1 tbsp chopped walnuts
- ½ tsp vanilla extract
- ¼ tsp cinnamon
- 1 tsp monk fruit sweetener

Serv.: 2

Method of Cooking: Freezing

Procedure:

Blend frozen banana, almond milk, vanilla extract, cinnamon, and monk fruit sweetener until smooth. Stir in chopped walnuts. Transfer to a container and freeze for at least 2 hours. Serve chilled.

N.V.: (per serving) Cal. 150 | Fat 6g | Carb. 18g | Prot. 3g

TOASTED ALMOND & COCONUT MACAROONS

P.T.: 5 minutes (preparation), 15 minutes (cooking)

Ingr.:
- ½ cup unsweetened shredded coconut
- 1 large egg white
- 1 tbsp chopped toasted almonds
- 1 tbsp monk fruit sweetener
- ½ tsp vanilla extract
- ¼ tsp salt

Serv.: 2

Method of Cooking: Baking

Procedure:

Preheat oven to 325°F. In a bowl, whisk egg white until frothy, then fold in shredded coconut, toasted almonds, monk fruit sweetener, vanilla extract, and salt. Form small mounds and place on a parchment-lined baking sheet. Bake for 15 minutes until golden brown. Let cool before serving.

N.V.: (per serving) Cal. 130 | Fat 10g | Carb. 6g | Prot. 3g

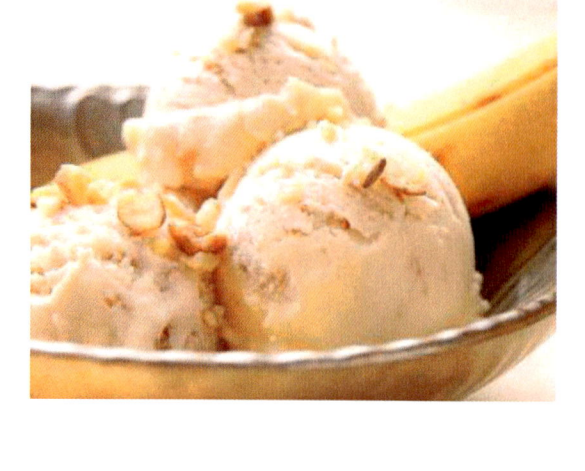

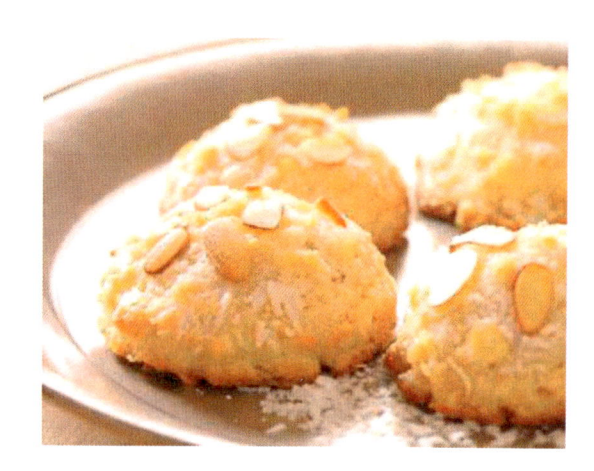

STRAWBERRY & BASIL GREEK YOGURT PARFAIT

P.T.: 5 minutes (preparation), 0 minutes (cooking)

Ingr.:
- ½ cup plain Greek yogurt
- ¼ cup fresh strawberries, sliced
- 1 tsp chopped fresh basil
- 1 tsp monk fruit sweetener
- ½ tsp vanilla extract
- 1 tbsp crushed walnuts

Serv.: 2

Method of Cooking: No-cook

Procedure:

In a bowl, mix Greek yogurt, monk fruit sweetener, and vanilla extract until smooth. Layer yogurt with sliced strawberries and chopped basil in serving cups. Sprinkle with crushed walnuts before serving.

N.V.: (per serving) Cal. 150 | Fat 7g | Carb. 10g | Prot. 10g

LOW-CARB CHEESECAKE WITH ALMOND CRUST

P.T.: 10 minutes (preparation), 25 minutes (cooking)

Ingr.:
- ½ cup almond flour
- 1 tbsp unsalted butter, melted
- ½ cup cream cheese, softened
- 1 tbsp monk fruit sweetener
- 1 large egg
- ½ tsp vanilla extract

Serv.: 2

Method of Cooking: Baking

Procedure:

Preheat oven to 350°F. In a bowl, mix almond flour and melted butter, then press into a small greased baking dish to form a crust. In another bowl, whisk cream cheese, monk fruit sweetener, egg, and vanilla extract until smooth. Pour over the crust and bake for 25 minutes. Let cool before serving.

N.V.: (per serving) Cal. 220 | Fat 18g | Carb. 6g | Prot. 8g

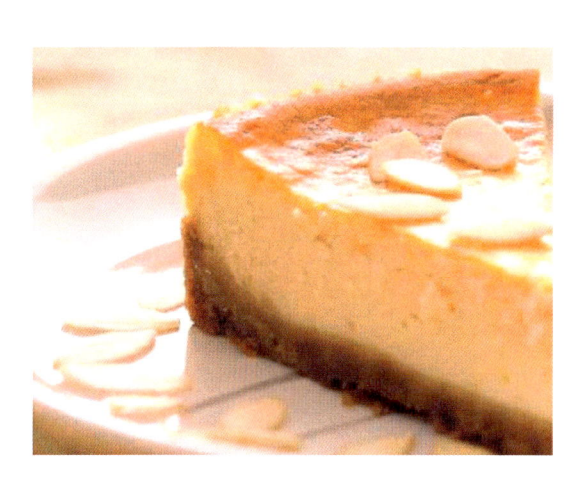

Chapter 7: Smart Snacks to Keep Your Energy Up Between Meals

SPICY ROASTED CHICKPEAS WITH PAPRIKA

P.T.: 5 minutes (preparation), 20 minutes (cooking)

Ingr.:
- ½ cup canned chickpeas, drained and rinsed
- 1 tbsp olive oil
- ½ tsp smoked paprika
- ¼ tsp garlic powder
- ¼ tsp salt
- ¼ tsp black pepper

Serv.: 2

Method of Cooking: Roasting

Procedure:

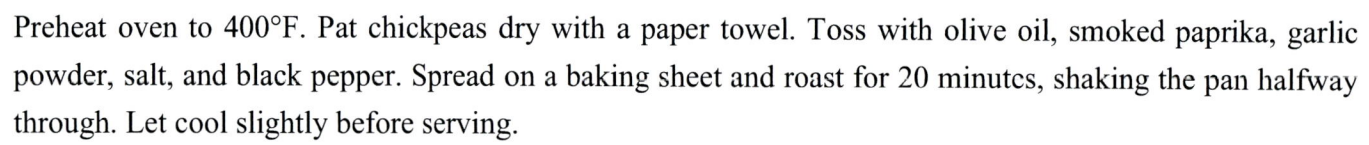

Preheat oven to 400°F. Pat chickpeas dry with a paper towel. Toss with olive oil, smoked paprika, garlic powder, salt, and black pepper. Spread on a baking sheet and roast for 20 minutcs, shaking the pan halfway through. Let cool slightly before serving.

N.V.: (per serving) Cal. 140 | Fat 7g | Carb. 14g | Prot. 5g

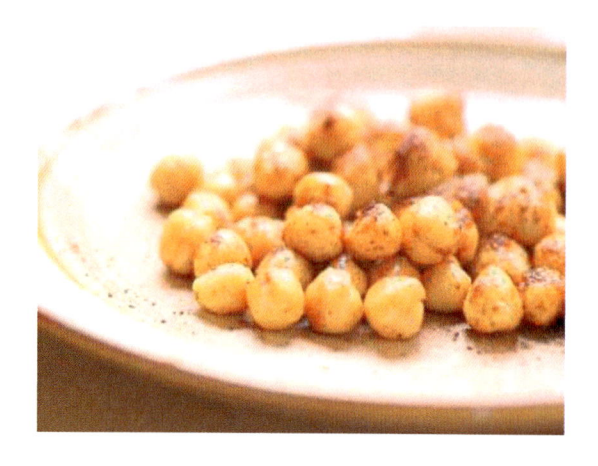

GREEK YOGURT & CUCUMBER DIP WITH WHOLE GRAIN CRACKERS

P.T.: 5 minutes (preparation), 0 minutes (cooking)

Ingr.:
- ½ cup plain Greek yogurt
- ¼ cup diced cucumber
- 1 tsp lemon juice
- ¼ tsp dried dill
- ¼ tsp garlic powder
- 4 whole grain crackers

Serv.: 2

Method of Cooking: No-cook

Procedure:

In a bowl, mix Greek yogurt, cucumber, lemon juice, dried dill, and garlic powder until well combined. Serve chilled with whole grain crackers.

N.V.: (per serving) Cal. 120 | Fat 3g | Carb. 12g | Prot. 8g

ALMOND BUTTER & CELERY STICKS WITH CHIA SEEDS

P.T.: 5 minutes (preparation), 0 minutes (cooking)

Ingr.:
- 2 celery stalks, cut into sticks
- 2 tbsp almond butter
- 1 tsp chia seeds
- ¼ tsp cinnamon
- 1 tsp monk fruit sweetener
- ¼ tsp vanilla extract

Serv.: 2

Method of Cooking: No-cook

Procedure:

Spread almond butter evenly over celery sticks. Sprinkle with chia seeds, cinnamon, monk fruit sweetener, and vanilla extract. Serve immediately.

N.V.: (per serving) Cal. 160 | Fat 12g | Carb. 8g | Prot. 5g

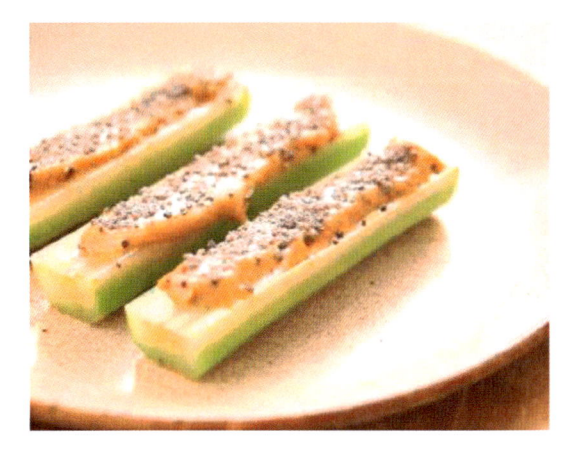

HARD-BOILED EGGS WITH AVOCADO & HOT SAUCE

P.T.: 10 minutes (preparation), 10 minutes (cooking)

Ingr.:

- 2 large eggs
- ½ small avocado, mashed
- ¼ tsp salt
- ¼ tsp black pepper
- ¼ tsp smoked paprika
- ½ tsp hot sauce

Serv.: 2

Method of Cooking: Boiling

Procedure:

Place eggs in a saucepan and cover with water. Bring to a boil, then simmer for 10 minutes. Remove eggs and place in ice water. Once cooled, peel and slice in half. Top with mashed avocado, salt, black pepper, smoked paprika, and a drizzle of hot sauce.

N.V.: (per serving) Cal. 180 | Fat 14g | Carb. 4g | Prot. 10g

SUGAR-FREE TRAIL MIX WITH NUTS & DARK CHOCOLATE BITS

P.T.: 5 minutes (preparation), 0 minutes (cooking)

Ingr.:

- 2 tbsp almonds
- 2 tbsp walnuts
- 1 tbsp pumpkin seeds
- 1 tbsp unsweetened dark chocolate chips
- ¼ tsp cinnamon
- ¼ tsp sea salt

Serv.: 2

Method of Cooking: No-cook

Procedure:

In a bowl, mix almonds, walnuts, pumpkin seeds, dark chocolate chips, cinnamon, and sea salt until well combined. Store in an airtight container or serve immediately.

N.V.: (per serving) Cal. 190 | Fat 14g | Carb. 8g | Prot. 5g

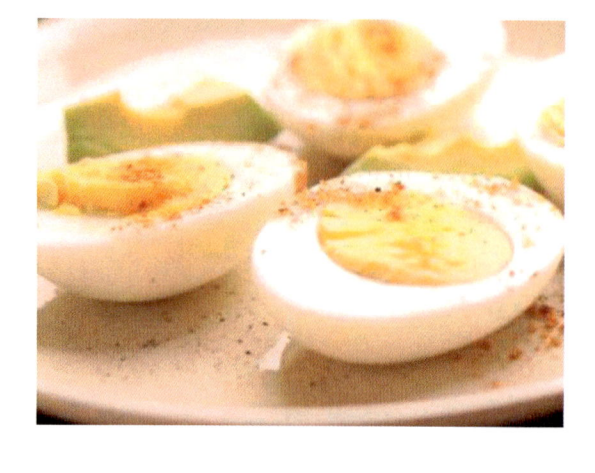

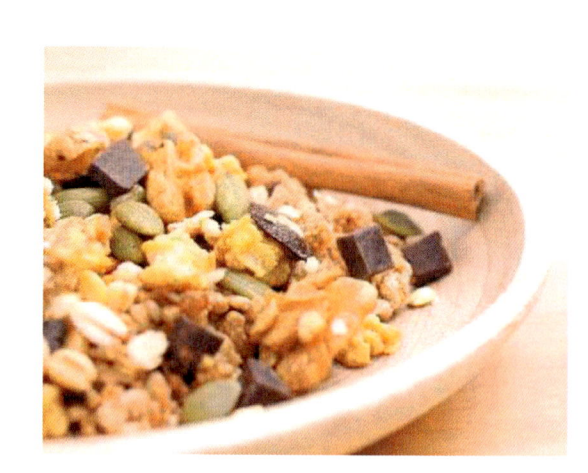

BAKED ZUCCHINI CHIPS WITH PARMESAN

P.T.: 5 minutes (preparation), 15 minutes (cooking)

Ingr.:
- 1 small zucchini, thinly sliced
- 1 tbsp olive oil
- 1 tbsp grated Parmesan cheese
- ¼ tsp garlic powder
- ¼ tsp black pepper
- ¼ tsp salt

Serv.: 2

Method of Cooking: Baking

Procedure:

Preheat oven to 375°F. Toss zucchini slices with olive oil, garlic powder, black pepper, and salt. Spread on a parchment-lined baking sheet. Sprinkle with Parmesan cheese and bake for 15 minutes until crisp. Serve warm.

N.V.: (per serving) Cal. 130 | Fat 9g | Carb. 7g | Prot. 4g

COTTAGE CHEESE & BERRIES WITH FLAXSEEDS

P.T.: 5 minutes (preparation), 0 minutes (cooking)

Ingr.:
- ½ cup cottage cheese
- ¼ cup fresh mixed berries
- 1 tsp ground flaxseeds
- 1 tsp monk fruit sweetener
- ½ tsp vanilla extract
- ¼ tsp cinnamon

Serv.: 2

Method of Cooking: No-cook

Procedure:

In a bowl, mix cottage cheese, monk fruit sweetener, vanilla extract, and cinnamon until smooth. Top with fresh berries and sprinkle with flaxseeds. Serve chilled.

N.V.: (per serving) Cal. 140 | Fat 5g | Carb. 10g | Prot. 12g

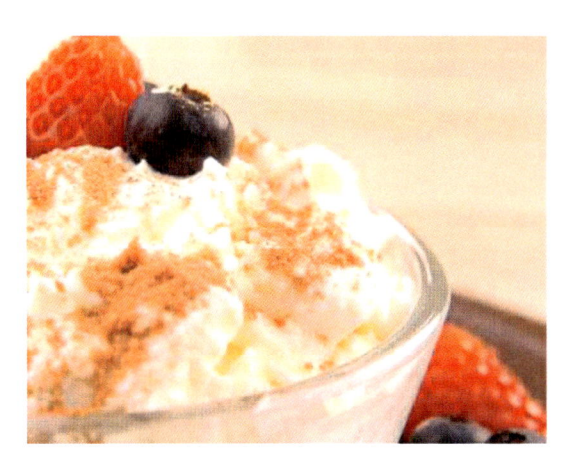

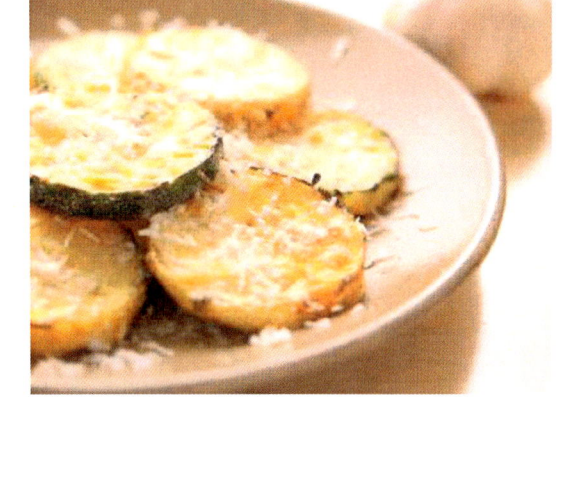

CUCUMBER & TURKEY ROLL-UPS WITH MUSTARD

P.T.: 5 minutes (preparation), 0 minutes (cooking)

Ingr.:
- 4 thin slices of turkey breast
- ½ small cucumber, julienned
- 1 tsp Dijon mustard
- 1 tsp olive oil
- ¼ tsp black pepper
- ¼ tsp dried oregano

Serv.: 2

Method of Cooking: No-cook

Procedure:

Spread Dijon mustard on turkey slices. Place julienned cucumber on each slice, roll up tightly, and secure with toothpicks. Drizzle with olive oil, sprinkle with black pepper and oregano, and serve immediately.

N.V.: (per serving) Cal. 110 | Fat 4g | Carb. 3g | Prot. 14g

ROASTED PUMPKIN SEEDS WITH SEA SALT & CINNAMON

P.T.: 5 minutes (preparation), 10 minutes (cooking)

Ingr.:
- ¼ cup raw pumpkin seeds
- 1 tsp olive oil
- ¼ tsp sea salt
- ¼ tsp cinnamon
- ¼ tsp smoked paprika
- ¼ tsp black pepper

Serv.: 2

Method of Cooking: Roasting

Procedure:

Preheat oven to 350°F. Toss pumpkin seeds with olive oil, sea salt, cinnamon, smoked paprika, and black pepper. Spread on a baking sheet and roast for 10 minutes until golden and fragrant. Let cool before serving.

N.V.: (per serving) Cal. 140 | Fat 10g | Carb. 4g | Prot. 6g

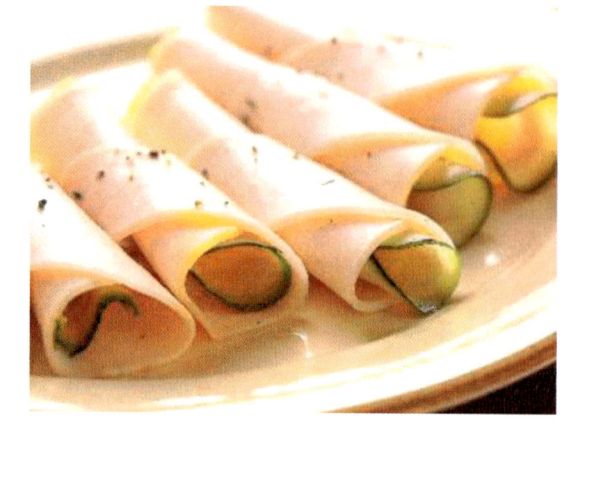

MINI BELL PEPPERS STUFFED WITH HUMMUS

P.T.: 5 minutes (preparation), 0 minutes (cooking)

Ingr.:
- 4 mini bell peppers, halved and deseeded
- ¼ cup hummus
- 1 tsp lemon juice
- ¼ tsp paprika
- ¼ tsp black pepper
- ¼ tsp sea salt

Serv.: 2

Method of Cooking: No-cook

Procedure:

Spoon hummus into each mini bell pepper half. Drizzle with lemon juice and sprinkle with paprika, black pepper, and sea salt. Serve immediately.

N.V.: (per serving) Cal. 120 | Fat 6g | Carb. 10g | Prot. 4g

ALMOND FLOUR CHEDDAR CRACKERS

P.T.: 5 minutes (preparation), 12 minutes (cooking)

Ingr.:
- ½ cup almond flour
- ¼ cup shredded cheddar cheese
- 1 tbsp unsalted butter, melted
- ¼ tsp garlic powder
- ¼ tsp sea salt
- ¼ tsp black pepper

Serv.: 2

Method of Cooking: Baking

Procedure:

Preheat oven to 350°F. In a bowl, mix almond flour, shredded cheddar, melted butter, garlic powder, sea salt, and black pepper until a dough forms. Roll out the dough and cut into small squares. Place on a parchment-lined baking sheet and bake for 12 minutes until golden and crispy. Let cool before serving.

N.V.: (per serving) Cal. 160 | Fat 12g | Carb. 5g | Prot. 6g

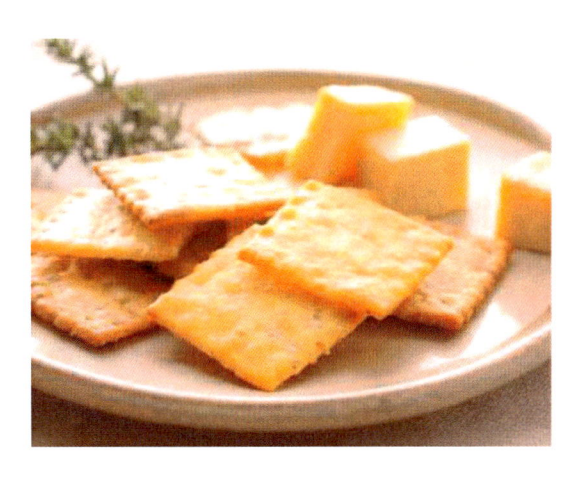

CHIA & COCONUT PROTEIN BITES

P.T.: 5 minutes (preparation), 0 minutes (cooking)

Ingr.:
- ¼ cup unsweetened shredded coconut
- 1 tbsp chia seeds
- 1 tbsp almond butter
- 1 tsp monk fruit sweetener
- ½ tsp vanilla extract
- 1 tsp water

Serv.: 2

Method of Cooking: No-cook, refrigeration

Procedure:

In a bowl, mix shredded coconut, chia seeds, almond butter, monk fruit sweetener, vanilla extract, and water until well combined. Shape into small balls and refrigerate for at least 20 minutes before serving.

N.V.: (per serving) Cal. 140 | Fat 10g | Carb. 6g | Prot. 4g

SMOKED SALMON & CREAM CHEESE CUCUMBER BITES

P.T.: 5 minutes (preparation), 0 minutes (cooking)

Ingr.:
- ½ small cucumber, sliced into rounds
- 2 oz smoked salmon
- 2 tbsp cream cheese
- ¼ tsp dried dill
- ¼ tsp black pepper
- 1 tsp lemon juice

Serv.: 2

Method of Cooking: No-cook

Procedure:

Spread cream cheese on cucumber slices. Top each with smoked salmon, a sprinkle of dried dill and black pepper, and a drizzle of lemon juice. Serve immediately.

N.V.: (per serving) Cal. 130 | Fat 8g | Carb. 4g | Prot. 10g

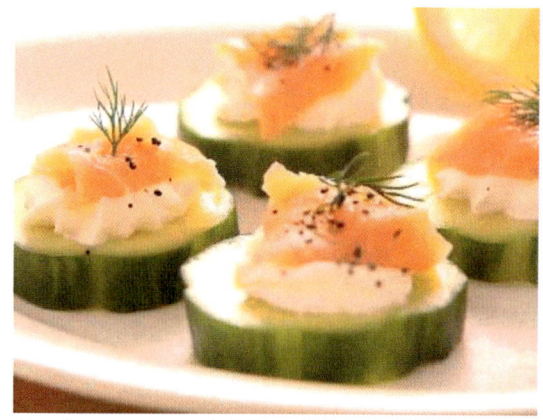

SUGAR-FREE PEANUT BUTTER PROTEIN BARS

P.T.: 5 minutes (preparation), 15 minutes (refrigeration)

Ingr.:
- ¼ cup natural peanut butter
- 2 tbsp almond flour
- 1 tbsp ground flaxseeds
- 1 tsp monk fruit sweetener
- ½ tsp vanilla extract
- 1 tbsp unsweetened almond milk

Serv.: 2

Method of Cooking: No-cook, refrigeration

Procedure:

In a bowl, mix peanut butter, almond flour, flaxseeds, monk fruit sweetener, vanilla extract, and almond milk until a dough forms. Press into a small dish and refrigerate for at least 15 minutes. Slice into bars and serve.

N.V.: (per serving) Cal. 180 | Fat 14g | Carb. 6g | Prot. 7g

SAUTÉED MUSHROOMS & SPINACH ON WHOLE GRAIN TOAST

P.T.: 5 minutes (preparation), 8 minutes (cooking)

Ingr.:
- ½ cup sliced mushrooms
- 1 cup fresh spinach
- 1 tsp olive oil
- ¼ tsp garlic powder
- ¼ tsp black pepper
- 2 slices whole grain toast

Serv.: 2

Method of Cooking: Sautéing

Procedure:

Heat olive oil in a skillet over medium heat. Sauté mushrooms for 5 minutes until tender. Stir in spinach, garlic powder, and black pepper, cooking for another 3 minutes until wilted. Spoon mixture onto whole grain toast and serve warm.

N.V.: (per serving) Cal. 160 | Fat 7g | Carb. 18g | Prot. 6g

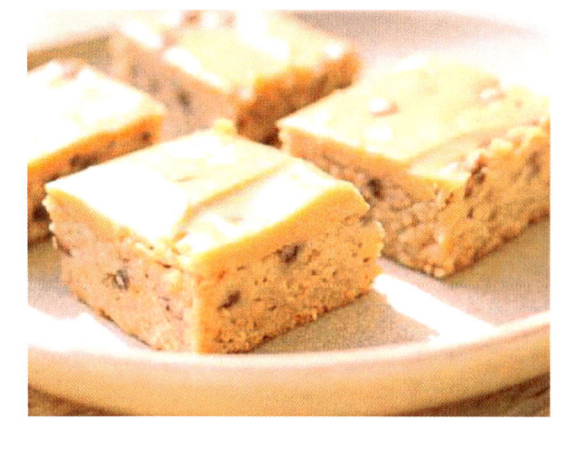

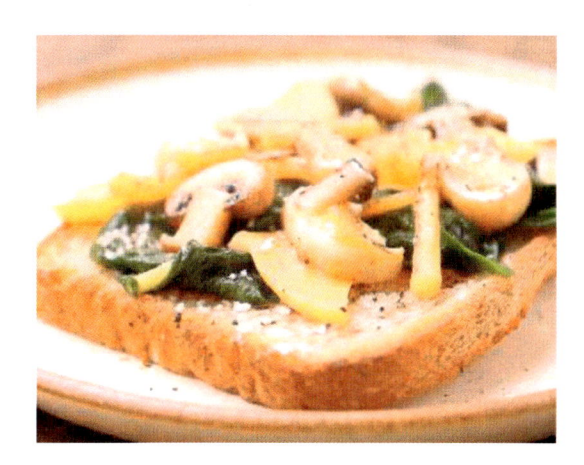

Conclusion

Managing diabetes through nutrition isn't about short-term fixes or strict diets—it's about creating a lifestyle that supports long-term health while still allowing for enjoyment. The key to lasting success lies in consistency, thoughtful planning, and a mindset that sees food as a tool for well-being rather than a limitation. Small, intentional choices add up, shaping a future of better energy, stability, and confidence in your health.

How to Maintain Long-Term Success with Your Diabetic-Friendly Diet

Sustaining a diabetic-friendly diet isn't about perfection; it's about persistence. The goal isn't to follow a rigid set of rules but to develop habits that feel natural, flexible, and enjoyable enough to last a lifetime. Making this way of eating a permanent part of daily life requires a balance between structure and adaptability—knowing when to stick to the plan and when to make adjustments without losing sight of the bigger picture.

Food choices should feel like second nature, not a constant source of decision fatigue. The key is consistency without monotony. Relying on a set of go-to meals can simplify daily eating, but variation keeps the experience satisfying. Rotating ingredients, exploring new flavors, and making small tweaks prevent burnout while ensuring a well-rounded intake of nutrients. A diet that becomes too repetitive often leads to frustration, while one that allows room for creativity and enjoyment is easier to sustain.

Life rarely follows a predictable routine, and neither do eating patterns. There will be days when schedules shift, when access to preferred foods is limited, or when temptations arise. Long-term success depends on resilience, not rigidity. The ability to make the best possible choice in any given situation—rather than feeling derailed by a single meal—determines whether healthy eating remains a lifelong practice or a temporary effort. When setbacks happen, as they inevitably will, the focus should be on regaining balance rather than dwelling on missteps. One indulgence doesn't undo progress, but an all-or-nothing mindset can.

Satisfaction plays a major role in adherence. A diet that feels restrictive is difficult to maintain, while one that prioritizes flavor and enjoyment naturally encourages consistency. Adjusting recipes to match personal taste preferences, incorporating favorite ingredients in a mindful way, and savoring meals instead of viewing them as obligations reinforce positive associations with eating well. The more enjoyable a meal plan is, the less willpower is required to stick with it.

Social situations, dining out, and travel can all present challenges, but they don't have to disrupt progress. Making informed choices in these settings comes down to awareness and preparation. Understanding how to modify meals, recognizing hidden sources of sugar and excess carbohydrates, and maintaining portion control in restaurants make it possible to enjoy meals without sacrificing stability. Developing strategies for these moments ensures that a single event doesn't spiral into long-term unhealthy patterns.

Over time, maintaining a diabetic-friendly diet becomes less about conscious effort and more about instinct. Cravings shift, preferences evolve, and the benefits of stable blood sugar—better energy, clearer thinking, fewer health concerns—reinforce the commitment to staying on track. The key to long-term success isn't in never straying from the plan, but in always finding a way back to it. The more these habits become part of daily life, the easier it is to maintain health without feeling like it requires constant sacrifice.

The Benefits of Consistency and Planning for Your Health

Health isn't built in a single meal, a single workout, or a single choice. It's the product of hundreds of small, intentional decisions made day after day. When it comes to managing diabetes, consistency isn't just helpful—it's essential. The body thrives on stability, and blood sugar control depends on maintaining balance over time. Erratic eating patterns, skipping meals, or switching between restrictive and indulgent phases create internal chaos, making it harder for the body to regulate glucose effectively. A steady, well-planned approach allows blood sugar levels to remain predictable, reducing the likelihood of sudden crashes or dangerous spikes.

Planning ahead removes the uncertainty that often leads to poor decisions. Without a plan, hunger dictates choices, and when blood sugar drops, the body craves quick fixes—processed snacks, sugary treats, or oversized portions of carbohydrates. Having structured meals in place prevents this from happening. When food is already prepared or ingredients are readily available, making a balanced choice becomes effortless. The more meals that align with health goals, the less impact occasional deviations have.

Beyond blood sugar control, consistency supports overall well-being. When meals are predictable and nutrient-dense, energy levels remain steady throughout the day. Mental clarity improves, and fatigue becomes less frequent. The digestive system functions more efficiently, and inflammation—often exacerbated by erratic eating habits—stays under control. Over time, maintaining a regular eating schedule strengthens the body's metabolic rhythm, reinforcing insulin sensitivity and reducing the strain on vital organs.

The benefits of planning extend beyond the plate. Thoughtful preparation simplifies grocery shopping, eliminates food waste, and reduces stress around mealtime. Instead of scrambling to find something to eat, meals become intentional, allowing for better portion control and nutrient balance. Planning also fosters a sense of control, removing the guesswork and anxiety that often accompany dietary changes. When a system is in place, eating well feels less like an effort and more like a habit.

Maintaining consistency doesn't mean never enjoying spontaneous moments. Life happens—social events, celebrations, unexpected schedule changes. The difference is that a structured foundation makes it easier to adapt without completely losing balance. When the majority of meals support long-term health, occasional indulgences have minimal impact. The key is to always return to the established routine rather than letting one deviation lead to a downward spiral.

Success isn't about never straying from the plan; it's about always having a plan to return to. Each balanced meal reinforces the next, each day of thoughtful eating makes the habit stronger. Over time, these choices add up, not just in better blood sugar control but in improved energy, greater confidence, and a stronger, more resilient body. The path to better health isn't about being perfect—it's about being consistent.

Encouragement for Your Ongoing Journey to Better Health

Every meaningful change starts with a single decision. The choice to take control of health, to make mindful food selections, to create habits that support well-being—it all begins with the realization that you have more power over your body than you may have been led to believe. Diabetes may require attention, but it does not have to dictate your life. Food is not the enemy. It is a tool, a resource, and, when used correctly, a powerful means of regaining strength, stability, and confidence in your health.

The road ahead will not always be straightforward. There will be moments when progress feels effortless, and others when frustration creeps in. Cravings will challenge discipline, routines will be disrupted, and some days will feel harder than others. But one meal, one misstep, one moment of doubt does not erase everything you have built. Your body responds to the patterns you create over time, not to occasional detours. What matters is that you always find your way back to the foundation you have built.

The most lasting transformations come from small, consistent steps. No single change is too minor to make a difference. Each meal that supports balanced blood sugar is a victory. Every time you choose a nutrient-dense ingredient over a processed one, you reinforce habits that protect your health. A well-prepared meal, a strategic grocery trip, a mindful portion size—these are not restrictions; they are investments in a future where you feel stronger, more energized, and in control.

Your body is always adapting, always responding to the choices you make. The way you eat today shapes how you will feel tomorrow. Energy levels, mobility, mental clarity, and long-term health outcomes are all within your influence. With every nourishing meal, you are giving your body the tools it needs to function at its best. The changes you implement today are not just about preventing complications—they are about improving quality of life. They are about waking up feeling refreshed, moving without discomfort, and engaging in daily activities with confidence.

You are not alone in this. Countless others are on the same journey, making the same adjustments, learning how to navigate a lifestyle that prioritizes health without sacrificing the joy of eating. Support can come from many places—friends, family, medical professionals, or even your own self-discipline. The important thing is to recognize that every effort you make adds up.

This is not about following a perfect plan without deviation. It is about developing a way of eating that supports both your health and your happiness. Every choice you make has value, every effort you put in moves you forward. No matter where you are in your journey, the most important step is always the next one. Keep going. Your future self will thank you.

Scan the QR code to access your free bonus!

Made in the USA
Las Vegas, NV
18 April 2025